thebowentechnique
the inside story

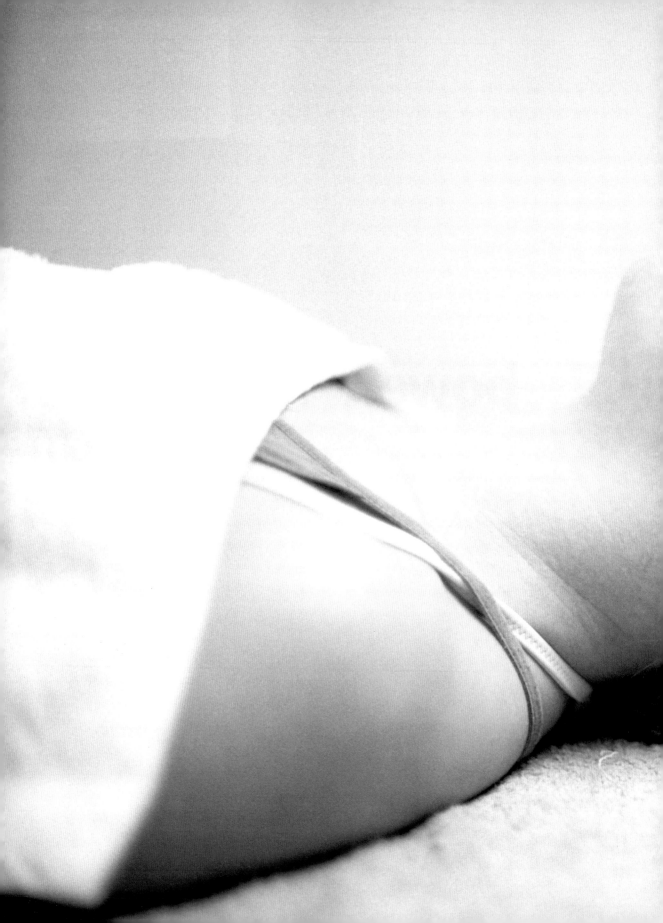

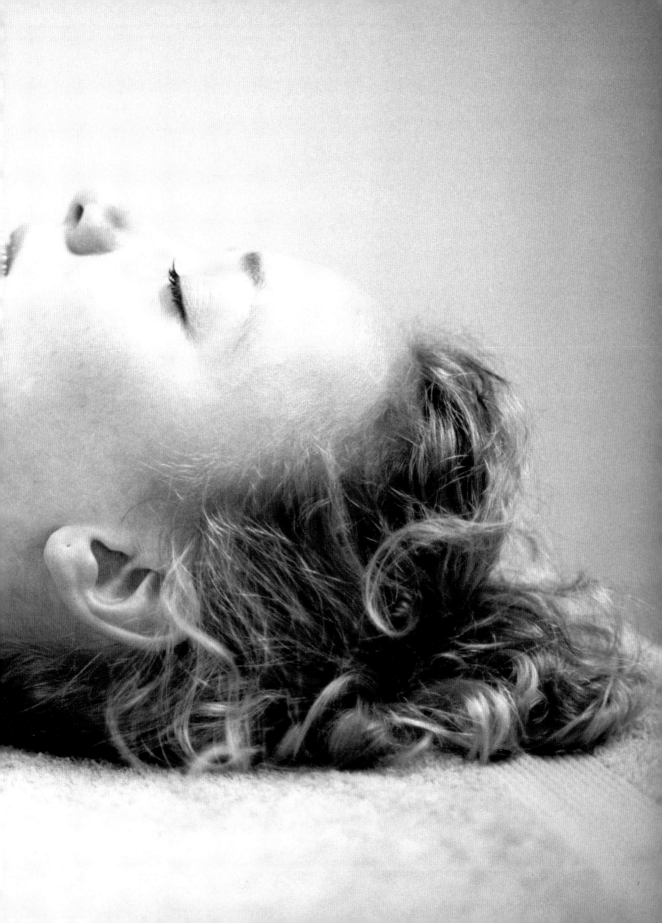

The Bowen Technique - The Inside Story

First published in Great Britain in 2007 by CYMA Ltd, Dorset, UK

www.cyma.org.uk   www.therapy-training.com

ISBN 978-0-9557063-0-1

British Library Cataloguing-in-Publication Data
A CIP record for this book is available from the British Library

Designed and typeset by RadioTrain Ltd, Bristol, UK
www.radiotrain.com

Printed & bound by Butler & Tanner, Somerset, UK
www.butlerandtanner.com

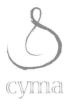

cyma

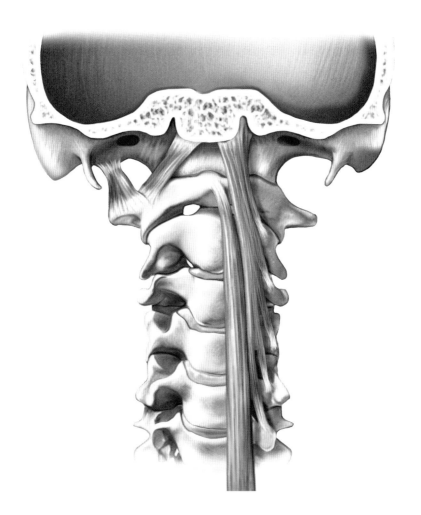

Credits

Illustrations on pages 10, 12, 13, 22, 23, 39, 68, 69, 74, 78, 81, 82, 84, 87, 97, 99, 112, 114, 121, 123, 127, 128, 131, 140, 143, 161, 162, 165, 253

Photography on pages 6, 48, 53, 56, 67, 71, 73, 77, 82, 83, 85, 86, 88, 100, 106, 111, 115, 118, 120, 122, 125, 126, 127, 128, 132, 134, 138, 140, 141, 144, 148, 170, 192, 238, 243, 248

Photograph of Tom Bowen courtesy Bowen Therapy Academy of Australia.

Image of Moro reflex on page 168 used with kind permission by the author from Goddard SA, 1996 *A teacher's window into the child's mind*. Fern Ridge Press. Eugene, OR. and Goddard SA, 2001 *Reflexes, learning and behavior*. Fern Ridge Press. Eugene.OR.

"Congratulations to John Wilks on a magnificent work. John's knowledge and understanding of how the Bowen Technique works is clearly manifested in this book. Posterity will acknowledge this work as an invaluable textbook for succeeding generations of Bowtech, the original Bowen Technique practitioners. Thank you John. Sincere appreciation."

Oswald Rentsch, Director, Bowen Therapy Academy of Australia.

"I highly recommend this authoritative book to all those who are interested in this most fascinating technique."

Michael M.Dooley, Consultant Obstetrician and Gynaecologist.

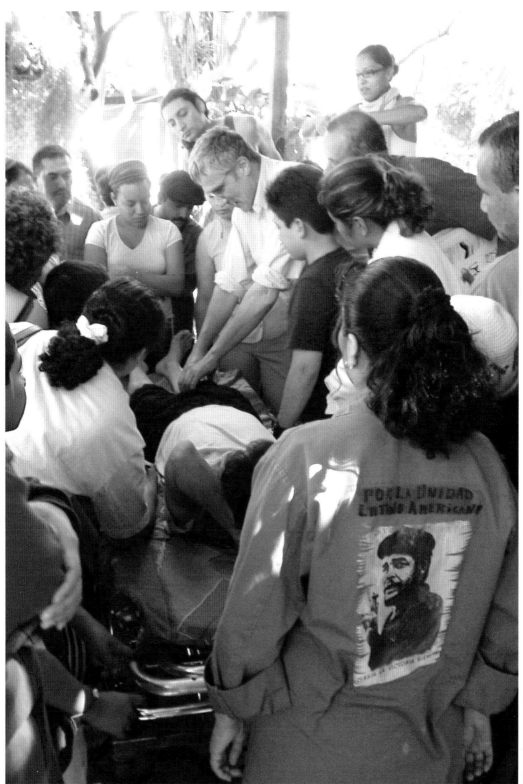

Contents

Preface 3

What are we doing?

1   What are we doing? 9

2   Fascia - Our Natural Communication System? 19

3   Embryological Development and the Uprising Midline 35

4   The Esoteric 43

Assessing the Client

5   Resources 51

6   What goes up must come down (and vice versa) 65

7   Orthopaedic Tests 77

8   Working with Chronic Pain and Facilitation 91

The Procedures

9   The Procedures 103

10   The Lower Body 111

11   The Upper Body 131

Fertility and Birth

12   Assisting Conception 151

13   Birth – First Impressions 159

Life after Treatment

14   What goes in must come out 173

15   Being Professional 179

16   Promote yourself! 187

The Therapeutic Relationship *by Su Fox*

17   Therapeutic Relationship Vignettes 195

18   The Importance of the Client – Practitioner Relationship 201

19   Self-care 209

20   The Practical Aspects of the Client - Practitioner Relationship 215

21   Unconscious Processes in the Therapeutic Relationship 229

Epilogue

22   Where do we go from here? 241

Appendices

A Note of Caution 251

Contact details 254

Ordering books by John Wilks 255
The Bowen Technique – The Inside Story
Understanding The Bowen Technique & Understanding Craniosacral Therapy

Bibliography 256

Reference text 260
The Acupuncture System and The Liquid Crystalline Collagen Fibres of the
Connective Tissues - Liquid Crystalline Meridians

References 268

Biography: *John Wilks* 273

Research References 275

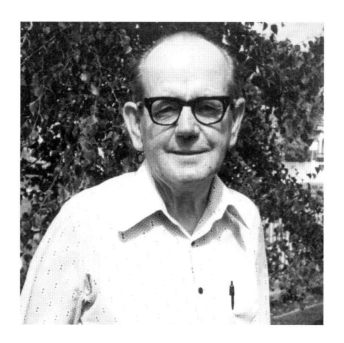

Thomas Ambrose Bowen
1916 – 1982

"I expect to pass through this world but once:
Any good thing therefore that I can do, or any kindness
that I can show to any fellow creature let me do it now.
Let me not defer or neglect it, for I shall not pass this way again."

Wilfred Whitten (John O'London)

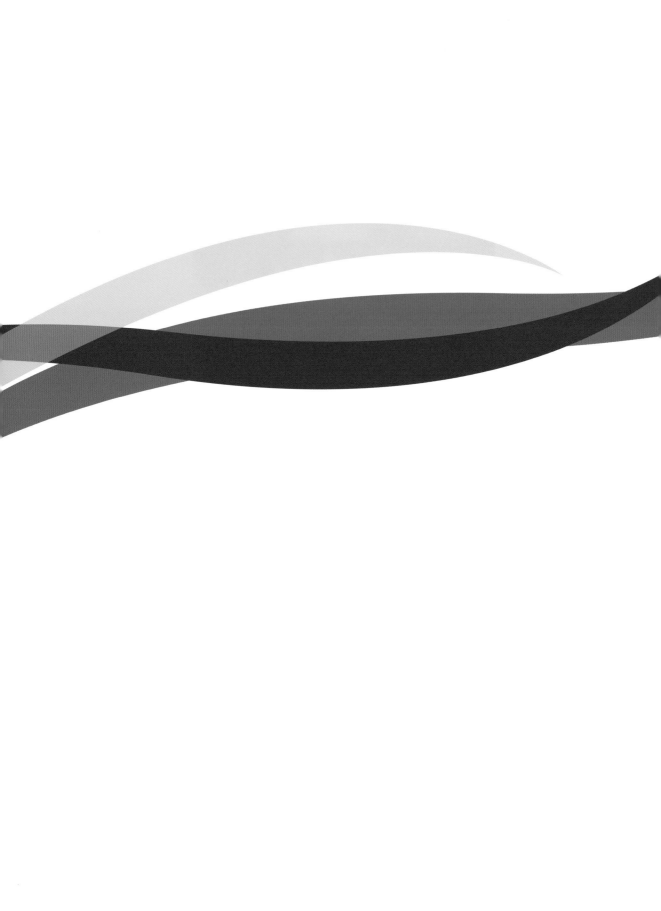

thebowentechnique
the inside story

John Wilks

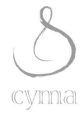

cyma

Preface

"A doctor who prescribes an identical treatment in two individuals and expects an identical development, may be properly classified as a social menace." - Lin Yutang.

This may seem like a strange quotation to introduce this book, given that nowadays most Bowen practitioners tend to follow strict formulae and appear to treat presenting symptoms in a similar way from patient to patient. However, it is clear that the originator of the work, Tom Bowen, rarely worked in this way and was constantly looking for the root cause of someone's condition, even if the symptoms were almost identical.

He developed his technique through impeccable observation of his clients, and indeed many seasoned and highly experienced osteopaths would ask for his opinion with patients they were finding difficult to treat. Tom Bowen's unerring ability to identify compensation patterns and what osteopaths would call 'lesions', made him legendary in his time and was in no small measure responsible for his outstanding success in treating such a wide range of conditions.

During the course of this book I would like to draw attention to the heart of this work, which is listening, observation and minimal intervention. Whatever anyone else who has their own ideas about this work says, it is very clear that Mr Bowen himself was the epitome of minimalism. For him, why perform five moves on a client when one will do? Especially when one will work better!

All those who worked with Tom Bowen or were treated by him commented on this highly unusual approach which seemed to go against the grain of thinking at the time. For a seasoned manipulator, the deeper the problem the more effort would be required on the part of the practitioner. For Tom Bowen the opposite was true, and the truth of this conviction is borne out by results not only in his own clinic in Geelong, Australia, but now in clinics across the globe.

There are other treatment approaches that share a similar

philosophy of 'less is more', along with the observation that there is an innate ability for the body to heal itself. In this philosophy of healing, often all that is needed is to 'listen' to the client's system in the right way and give it the smallest assistance possible for healing to take place at a deep level. The secret of the work is to step back and allow the body to do its work.

As Rollin Becker, an American cranial osteopath, used to say:

"When you are dealing with the highest known energy that's available, it doesn't want anyone interfering with what it's trying to do."

This 'highest known energy' is the fundamental basis of many healing traditions throughout the ages. Cranial osteopaths used to call it 'The Breath of Life', a term taken from the Old Testament to refer to the powerful organising forces inherent in nature and consciousness. In other healing traditions it is depicted as the caduceus, a powerful symbol that represents uprising healing forces orientated to the human midline which has strong overlays with the development of the embryo.

There is no doubt that we tap into some very primal organising forces in Bowen work and that Dr Still, the originator of osteopathy, recognised this as the fundamental principle when he was developing his work in the late 1800's. Both osteopathy and cranial osteopathy have a lot in common on a philosophical level with Tom Bowen's work, even if nowadays the original vision has been somewhat lost.

Dr Still would frequently say to his students:

"The first object of the physician is to find health – anyone can find disease."

If there is one motto that every Bowen practitioner should have on the wall of their clinic, this would be it. It describes our job perfectly. We are the health finders, the ghost-busters of the complementary healing world, whose job is to find that kernel of health, water it, feed it and allow it to grow.

The object of this book is to get back to the heart of this extraordinary work which was developed by a man who was undoubtedly a genius. Tom Bowen developed his vision with very little written down and very little explanation in his own words. It has been up to pioneers like Oswald Rentsch and others that were taught by Tom Bowen to explain his principles.

This book is the result of 12 years' observation of the effects of Mr Bowen's technique on thousands of clients. I know I am still only scratching the surface of this remarkable work, but it is obvious that its potential has hardly begun to be realised.

It is with immense gratitude that I dedicate this book to Oswald and Elaine Rentsch in the hope that it reflects the spirit of this work with the integrity that Tom Bowen showed to his clients and the people who worked with him.

This book would not have been possible without the generous help of Goff Rumbles and Damian Connop of RadioTrain, my beautiful partner Georgina Robinson who kindly laboured for hours over the proofs and did some of the drawings, Daniela B Larsen who bravely offered to be a model for the photos, my sons Naren Wilks who brought his supreme talent to the photos, and Lyndon who modelled for some of the photos. I would also like to thank Dr Mae Wan Ho, James Oschman, Sally Goddard Blythe and Katherine Ukleja who generously gave their assistance along with many of my Bowen colleagues, particularly Rick Minnery, Dr Claire Picken and Martin Grasby.

John Wilks
August 2007

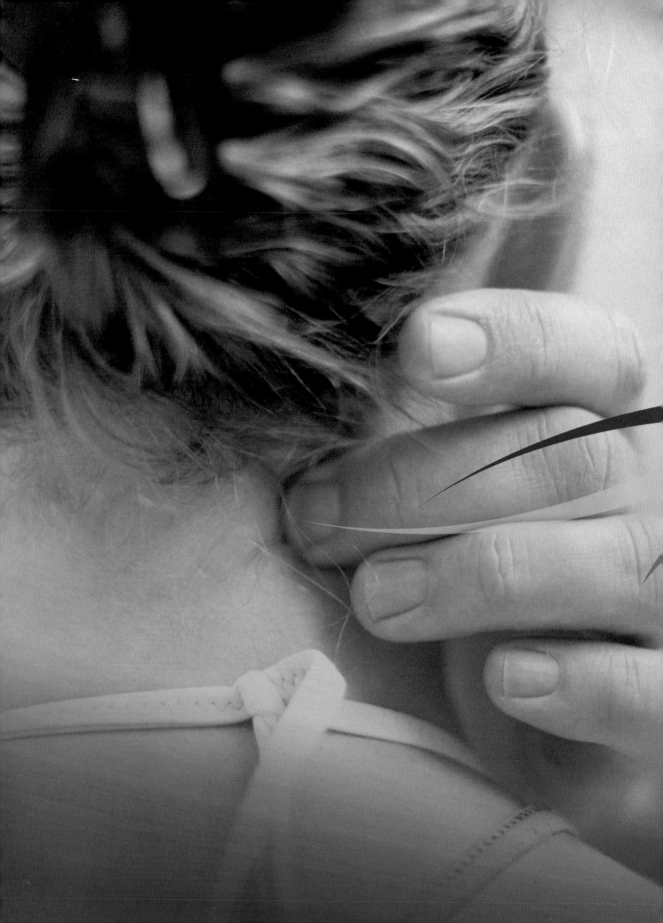

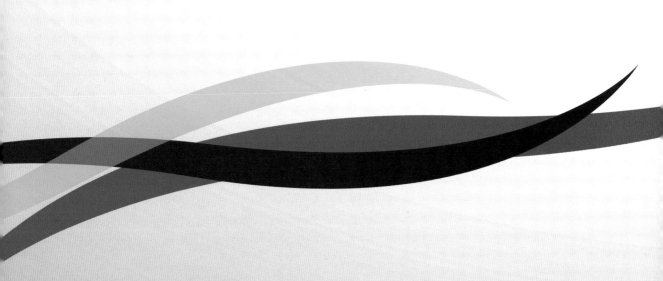

what are we doing?

Chapter 1

What are we doing?

The Bowen Technique involves very gentle but direct manipulation of the following structures in the body:

- Muscles
- Tendons
- Fascia
- Ligaments
- Joints
- Nerves

In a classic Bowen move one of these structures will be activated, in another possibly two or three at the same time, depending on where the move is being performed. However, a common thread is that all Bowen moves involve some sort of activation of fascia, as it envelops, or is integral to, all the above.

Mostly, Bowen moves are made directly on muscles themselves, over the 'belly' or centre of the muscle between its origin and insertion. Because almost all structures in the body are surrounded by fascia - thin, tough translucent sheets of fibrous material that contain, separate and allow free movement between the structures they envelop, it is inevitable that as a muscle is activated, the fascia that surrounds it, and is integral to it, is affected at the same time, albeit with slightly different physiological effects.

All structures that are activated during a Bowen treatment, whether skin, organs, joints or muscles, also have sensory nerves innervating them in order to give feedback to the spinal cord and the brain about the state of that particular structure – whether it is hot, cold, stretched, painful, etc.

Muscles are full of particular nerve receptors called muscle spindles which relay whether that muscle is stretched or not. With every movement we do, certain muscles contract which means that corresponding muscles have to extend. This activity is controlled at the level of the spinal cord and the brain.

Muscle spindles which lie alongside the tiny muscle fibres relay the state of the muscle in terms of stretch, and there are many, many of them within each muscle, depending on the degree of sensitivity required. The deep muscles of your neck have as many as 150 - 200 per gram of muscle tissue whereas the buttock, where less sensitivity is needed, only has about 50 per gram. Interestingly, the muscles on either side of the spine (the erector spinae muscles), which we work a lot in Bowen work, have exceptionally high levels of muscle spindles – around 200 – 500 per gram of muscle tissue.

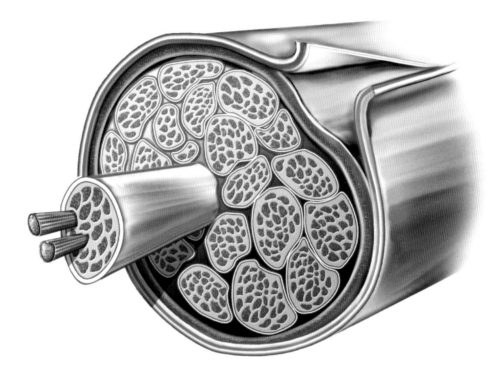

Sometimes we work closer to where the muscle attaches on to bone, on tendon effectively. Here we effect another feedback mechanism – the Golgi tendon organs that lie in the tendons themselves and are sensitive to resistance in the muscle and which dictate how much force is needed to lift something or resist an external force. This is useful to us in terms of our biceps, for example, being able to tell the difference between a rock and picking up our cup of coffee in the morning. Without Golgi tendons the coffee could easily end up over our shoulders!

The Golgi tendon organs have an interesting function in that they produce an inhibitory effect on both slow and fast twitch muscle fibres when the amplitude of the stretch becomes too severe. We use this function when we hold a strong Bowen challenge on a tendon (such as move 2 of the pelvic procedure), with the result that the muscle will begin to relax under our hands.

One way of explaining the work in physical terms is its effect on the nerves within muscles. Firstly, as a challenge is placed on a muscle, and the muscle is gently stretched, these stretch receptors begin to send sensory information along the nerve pathways to the spinal cord. The information that is fed back in this way depends on a complex interaction of different nerves – some fast acting (like mechanoreceptors) and some slow acting (like nociceptors).

During the day as one moves around these nerves send information many thousand times a second to the brain as to the status of individual muscles. The pathway is a little complicated. Initially, when the muscle spindles fire off in response to a lengthening in muscle, impulses are created which travel along the sensory nerves to the spinal cord.

In the adult, some of these sensory nerve pathways can be quite long. Take the foot, for example. Sensory information from the muscles, fascia, skin, joints and connective tissue travels along these sensory nerve pathways right up to the middle of the back (T12) before reaching the spinal cord. Once the impulses reach the spinal cord, some response happens in terms of a 'reflex' – i.e. a motor response can be initiated at this level which results in the muscles at the same level of the spinal cord (spinal segment) being contracted. This happens in the knee reflex test, when a gentle blow to the patella tendon creates a response in our quad muscles initiated by our femoral nerve.

Beyond this simple reflex, information is also shunted up towards the brain via the various spinal tracts in the spinal cord. These could be seen as the motorways of our central nervous system. Sensory spinal tracts ferry sensory information to the brain, whilst motor tracts transmit information back to muscles and organs in response to information received not only from our

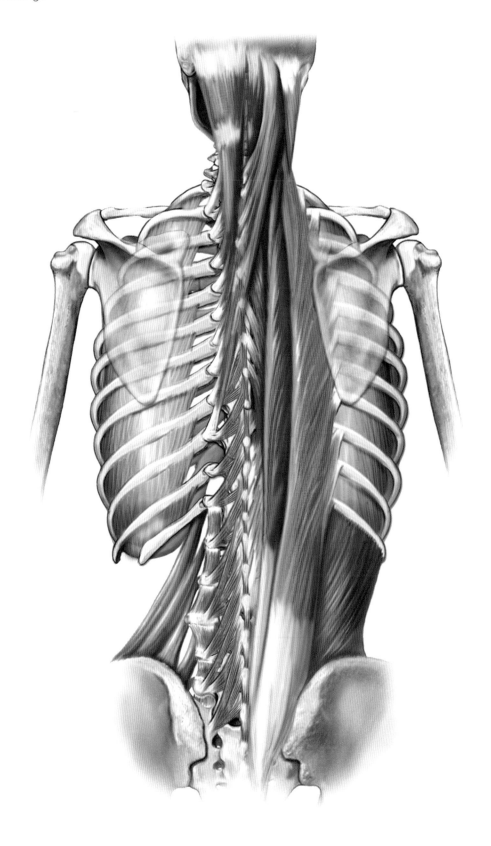

muscles, but also from our eyes and our organs of balance (our vestibular system).

Once this sensory information reaches the brain, it goes through a highly complex procedure where it is shunted backwards and forwards between various areas like the cerebellum, the basal ganglia, the reticular formation and the brain stem before being co-ordinated in the thalamus and sent back down the various motor nerve tracts to the muscles or organs that are innervated by motor nerves. At this level, sensory nerve activity outnumbers motor nerve activity by about three to one.

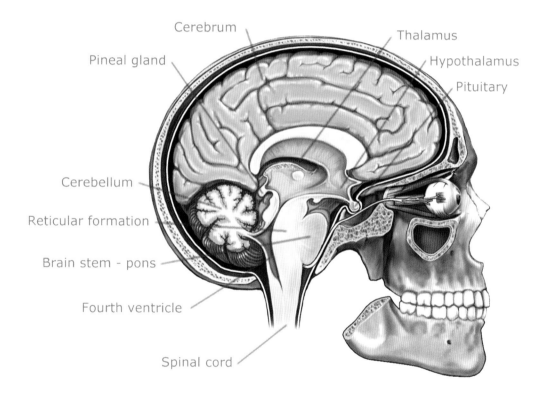

Cerebrum
Thalamus
Pineal gland
Hypothalamus
Pituitary
Cerebellum
Reticular formation
Brain stem - pons
Fourth ventricle
Spinal cord

What is interesting for us is that during a Bowen treatment, a stretch on the muscle is maintained for several seconds before the move itself is made. As this stretch is initiated, sensory information is sent via nerves to the spinal cord and then to these various areas of the brain. Research has shown that it takes around 90 seconds for muscles to respond to input in this way, something that is used in the osteopathic technique of strain-counterstrain. Whether Tom Bowen was aware of this when he insisted on leaving the body for two minutes between moves is not known, but the fact is that it is of vital importance in the process of allowing the body time to respond to the work.

Whilst awake and moving around, huge amounts of information from our muscles, tendons, joints, skin and fascia is being processed at any one time, but while we are lying down there is very little activity happening within this self-corrective system.

What seems then to be happening during a Bowen session is that the body is allowed to re-orient to a memory of a previously healthy state or an original blueprint of health. Because Bowen moves are made at key structural points in the body that the brain uses as natural reference points to determine its posture (a lot of these points refer back to significant structures embryologically and developmentally), therefore moves at these precise points have a huge effect on the way that the body holds itself.

A few factors are important. Firstly, if a Bowen therapist were to do many extraneous moves without pauses, the effect would be greatly minimised. This is why a favourite Bowen maxim is 'less is more'. Secondly, if the person is not relaxed or comfortable the primitive areas of the brain that are involved with the co-ordination of movement would not be able to 'hear' and process this distinct information to its benefit. It would be a bit like someone trying to listen to very precise instructions whilst a hammer drill was being used in the background or someone was speaking too quickly.

About 6 years ago I organised a conference in London and invited as a speaker Michel Odent, a pioneer in the natural birth movement. Whilst he was talking about the ideal condition for a mother to give birth, it occurred to me that there were clear parallels with a Bowen treatment.

He explained that the ideal situation for the mother was one in which there was as little interference to the mother's natural process as possible. Specifically, he cited certain activities which interrupted these processes by activating the cortex, the area of the brain more involved with conscious control:

1. Speaking to the patient, particularly if the conversation refers to something that is not in the patient's current field of sensation (for example, asking where they went on holiday or what their mother's maiden name is!)

2. Feeling cold

3. Feeling unsafe

4. Bright lights

Because it is important for the autonomic nervous system to begin to re-calibrate itself and for the corrective feedback mechanism between the various centres that control postural muscle relationships to go through this process free of external interruption, we can deduce that the ideal situation to conduct a Bowen session would be this:

1. No talking to the client unless it is related to physical sensation in the body in present time.

2. Keeping the client nice and warm. Usually if the practitioner is wearing anything thicker than a T-shirt then it will be too cold in the treatment room.

3. The client should feel safe. The fact that the practitioner conducts himself in a professional manner that maintains clear boundaries is crucial to the client's feelings of safety. Even what the practitioner is thinking (for example thinking that the client is particularly attractive or particularly unattractive will influence whether a client would feel safe or not). Draping the client appropriately will also help in making the client feel secure and able to relax.

4. Bright lights activate the cortex, so a dimmer in your treatment room is very helpful. Flourescent lights also have a contracting effect on smooth muscle (for example the muscles around the heart), so are particularly bad.

5. Music tends to have an activating effect on the mind and can have strong emotional resonances in the client. In any case, it is much better if the client can settle into their own sensation rather than be drawn into the emotional state of the music.

There are many other explanations as to how the technique works. It is clear that some of the points worked on relate to acupuncture meridians and trigger points. Therapists also often notice a response through their hands as they work, as though an electrical impulse is created as a result of a move. Tom Bowen used to describe how he used the information from these subtle impulses to read responses in the body as he was working.

In fact, these impulses are measurable – it has been shown that the creation of a stretch in the fascia does indeed initiate a small piezo-electrical charge. Studies in the USA have measured these and identified them as being created by the tiny collagen fibres which make up the bulk of fascia, and that these impulses have very powerful healing effects on the body.

Experiments have shown that artificially passing a low-level current of this type over a broken bone will greatly speed up repair but that the degree of current is crucial – too strong a current is counter-productive and will hinder repair. This of course has implications for us in terms of how much pressure we use with our Bowen moves – the greater the pressure, the stronger the electrical impulse created. It would be very interesting to do some research on the optimum pressure needed for optimal response on tissue. The implications for this are discussed in the next chapter.

Chapter 2

Fascia - Our Natural Communication System?

"The soul of man with all the streams of pure living water seems to dwell in the fascia of his body"

A.T. Still

An understanding of the nature and function of fascia is really crucial to becoming a good Bowen practitioner.

Fascia has extraordinary properties. It surrounds organs and other structures in the body such as muscles and it allows free movement and 'glide' between these structures as we move around.

You will have seen sheets of fascia – translucent sheets of connective tissue – when you prepare a chicken for the oven. In terms of its quality it is rather like a plastic shopping bag in that it retains its strength without stretching very much, but will tend to hold patterns if it is damaged or stressed.

Tom Bowen was intensely interested in fascia and would study carcasses of animals at his local abatoir to see how the fascia was structured in the body.

Fascia is made up primarily of collagen fibres. These are small hollow tubes filled with very fine fluid – similar to cerebro-spinal fluid which is very high in photons or light particles. Collagen is a protein which makes up around 70% of all the protein in connective tissue and is the most common protein in the animal kingdom. It also has unique properties in that water molecules are attracted to it and will stick to it in a very ordered way, a bit like scaffolding around a building.

This quality allows a high degree of fluidity in the fascia which is essential both for the free movement and glide (e.g between groups of mucles, or between organs) and also for effective intercellular communication. The degree of fluidity in the fascia is determined by use and hydration – gentle stretching is one of the best ways to encourage fluidity into the tissues.

Not only is drinking water important for the hydration of fascia, but also the quality of the water is crucial. In normal tap water, water molecules group together in about 10 – 12 whereas in more alkaline water (for example water that has been ionized, although there is some controversy around the advisability of drinking ionized water long-term) it groups in 5 – 6. The smaller grouping in alkaline water seems to be much more effective at ridding the body of toxins as it is able to pass more freely through the cell walls.

The structure of fascia is determined by its use. The collagen fibres orient themselves to the stress and structural loading imposed by standing, walking, sitting etc. In the baby, as it goes from crawling to standing, you can see the differing stress patterns that will be placed upon the myo-fascial system as this happens. These early movements of the baby are crucial in the development of the fascia and, particularly relevant to our work, the orientation of the collagen fibres.

One particularly important band of fascia that determines our posture is the ilio-tibial band up the sides of the leg. This is easy to palpate. If you feel around the seam of the trouser on the side of the leg you will feel a tough fibrous band. The patterns of stress imposed on this band are primarily vertical in a standing position, so that most collagen fibres within it lie in a superior/inferior orientation.

Effects on Fascia

The health of fascia is affected by several factors. Firstly, hydration is crucial to its effectiveness. Gentle stretching, such as yoga or Pilates, is excellent as it helps orient the collagen fibres within the fascia and also creates space for fluids around and within the cells.

Stretching fascia can be likened to applying force to metal – if one were to bend a metal bar too strongly or too fast it makes it brittle. If one bends it slowly then it encourages it to become more fluid and flexible. Stretching too forcefully can also create inflammation in the tissues which is counter-productive to recovery.

One of the problems with people who go to the gym, particularly if they are competitive in nature, is that it is so easy for them to damage themselves through inappropriate exercise. Individual muscle fibres are surrounded by fascia and when people do compressive exercise such as weights it is easy for them to tear. This is what gives the impression that muscles are being built up.

In reality, often the extra muscle bulk derives from a tearing and bunching up of the muscle fibres. This creates adhesions through the tissues and a lack of ability for the body to get rid of toxins.

At the other extreme, the average couch potato who does very little exercise (say who walks less than 20 minutes a day) will have a lot of congestion in their connective tissues. The lymphatic system depends on movement to do its job. Likewise, the orientation of the collagen fibres depends on use, and this orientation is crucial to the effectiveness of our work (see below).

Scars and operations will also affect fascia and can create 'breaks' in the fascial tracts. This can cause adhesions around a particular area and often several layers of fascia at once. For example, if one has a scar around the kidney area it will tend to restrict the free movement of the fascia surrounding the latissimus dorsi muscle. Because this muscle attaches on to the arm it will affect the ability to raise the arm.

You can see the effect of this yourself. In a standing position, place the palm of your hand flat under the opposite arm pit and press into the side of the body fairly firmly right onto the latissimus dorsi muscle. Now raise your arm up and outwards laterally from the body. As you do so you will feel a restriction through your latissimus muscle which will inhibit your ability to raise your arm.

There are many other examples like this – a caesarean scar may pull through the linea alba up towards the umbilicus, through to the pericardium around the heart and then through the pre-tracheal fascia in the front of the neck. If one looks at the various fascial 'trains' as described in Thomas Myer's book, *Anatomy Trains*, it is easy to see how restrictions in any of these fascial relationships will affect the whole.

I remember a few years ago treating a woman with extreme tightness through her hamstrings. She was a professional athlete and hurdling was one of her specialities. Over a few sessions, we proceeded to address the most obvious areas – working around the hamstrings, the sacrum and the knees, but to no avail. She then told me that she had broken bones in both her

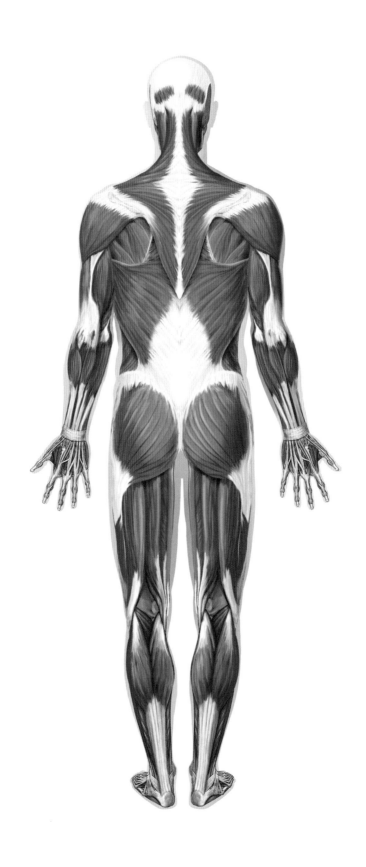

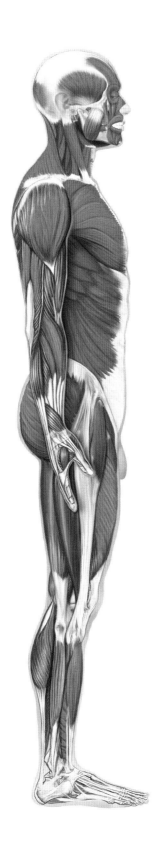

"Fascia...must be free at all parts to
receive and discharge all fluids,...
and eject all impurities, that health
may not be impaired by dead and
poisonous fluids. A knowledge of
the universal extent of the fascia
is imperative, and is one of the
greatest aids to the person who
seeks the causes of disease."
A. T. Still

feet at different times. Although the bones had repaired well, on examination, the plantar fascia in her feet were very tight.

I decided to do the 'hammer toes' procedure which involves a few moves over the plantar fascia. She had a very strong reaction on the couch and had to lie there for around 20 minutes. When she got up off the couch she instinctively wanted to test her range of movement by trying to touch her toes. She could easily get both palms flat on the ground without discomfort. Previously she had only been able to get her fingertips around 3 inches from the ground.

I was astounded by this result (as was she delighted) and I began to consider how this might be possible. It is clear that there is a direct fascial connection between the plantar fascia in the foot through the gastrocnemius to the hamstrings, but how did such a small release allow for such a massive increase in range of motion? I began to look more at the nature of fascia and new research into how it can hold patterns and communicate impulses.

The Secrets of Fascia

An important pioneer in research into the nature of connective tissue is Dr Mae Wan Ho. A scientist working in London, she has been an outspoken opponent of GM engineering of food. Her book *The Rainbow and the Worm* and research papers are available from her website at www.i-sis.org.uk

I have summarized the main implications of her work below. Extracts from a paper on the properties of connective tissue is published in the appendix with her permission.

Impulses

Impulses are created in the collagen fibres by very light pressure. Research in the USA has shown that stressing collagen fibres by applying gentle pressure creates a small electrical charge which has strong healing properties. It has been shown that crosswise stretching as is used in Bowen creates a stronger piezoelectric current than just pressing on it (such as might be used in Rofling) or going along the length of it (as might be used in massage). The fact that impulses can also be affected by heat might give a clue as to why we ask clients to avoid exposing themselves to extremes of hot or cold after a session.

Conductivity

The conductivity of collagen increases strongly depending on how hydrated it is. This means that the impulses we create during a treatment will travel much more effectively if the fascia is hydrated. This is probably why some people respond better to the treatment than others – babies, animals and those who practice yoga all will tend to have a much more hydrated and fluid system.

Amplification

Impulses created by Bowen moves will be amplified via the action of proteins in liquid crystals. Mae Wan describes fascia as essentially liquid crystaline in nature, in other words highly responsive to electrical charge and able to carry electrical impulses very fast (much faster than the central nervous system). Furthermore, fascia also responds as a single coherent system – a bit like a liquid crystal display that is used in televisions. In other words, the fascia will respond AS A WHOLE to a Bowen move, not just locally, and it will respond in large part directionally, determined by how the impulses travel through it. This in turn is determined by the orientation of the collagen fibres, which in turn is determined by use.

The directional effect of Bowen moves should not be over-estimated, however, as it is important to understand the effect of a Bowen move on the whole extra-cellular matrix which is not necessarily directional but global, even affecting the energy field some distance from the body. The cellular changes that Bowen invokes in the body are measurable not only by conventional microscopy but also by more subtle energetic measurements.

Changes in cells

Physiological changes occur in cells in response to impulses created through the collagen.

Tissue Memory

Liquid crystals hold 'memory' which has the capacity to register new experience. In other words, it holds patterns of experience but is also highly receptive to change initiated by directional electrical impulses. James Oschman has called this phenomenon 'somatic recall' and cites research by Stuart Hameroff which describes how micro-tubules in the connective tissue also hold memory. When they are subjected to pressure, as happens in a Bowen move, they radiate a field which releases held tissue memory patterns which can sometimes then become conscious recall memories in the client and even the practitioner.

Drugs

Conductivity along the lines of collagen fibres is adversely affected by certain substances, for example anaesthetics. Many Bowen practitioners will have noticed that it is much more difficult to get good results if a patient has had a cortisone injection, for example, or is taking muscle relaxants.

Cortisone in particular has a fairly devastating affect on fascia and tends to create areas of density and lack of fluidity in the system. Some practitioners have found that using homeopathic cortisone is helpful in counteracting the effects of this drug.

Pathways

Impulses will travel around 100 times more strongly along the orientation of the collagen fibres as opposed to other directions. Given that these fibres orient to lines of use and structural stress, it is easy to see where impulses will travel in the body.

For example, a move over the vastus lateralis tendon ('hit the lat') will travel up the ilio-tibial band over the gluteal fascia and up the erector spinae to the occiput. If there is no congestion, scar tissue, lack of fluidity or dehydration in the fascia then impulses will be amplified as they travel.

When one looks at the patterns of fascia in the body as described by Ida Rolf and Thomas Myers, one will see clearly defined 'trains' and layers which will determine how and where the impulses we create travel.

Fascia forms itself in layers that move one against another. This means that impulses (ie Bowen moves) created in areas where fascia overlap will affect all those layers. Otherwise they would only travel along one layer at a time.

In Bowen we sometimes perform moves where there is an overlap of layers of fascia. These moves tend to be very powerful because we affect several layers at once.

Take moves 3 & 4 in the neck, for example; not only do these moves go over two important lymph nodes (the sub-occipital nodes), but they also affect three muscles and layers of fascia simultaneously.

Moves 1 & 2 of BRM 1 are also interesting in this regard as they affect not only the ilio-lumbar fascia which has fibres that are quite diffuse, but also the erector spinae fascia which has a clear superior/inferior orientation.

There is a strong continuity of fascia throughout the body and it has a very clear differentiation front and back. Take, for example, the small moves that we do either side of the trachea in the upper respiratory procedure. These small moves may seem insignificant, but in fact they create an impulse that travels down the pre-tracheal fascia, continues to the pericardium which surrounds the heart, travels down the falciform ligament to the umbilicus and the linea alba to the pubis.

This of course will depend if we have put any 'stoppers' in beforehand. The lower respiratory moves on the front at the diaphragm can act as stoppers and inhibit the impulses travelling through the front fascia at this level. This can be very useful if we want to contain the work above or below the level of the diaphragm.

We use this principle when we do the thoracic procedure to address scoliosis. We can also use it to address the abdominal cavity if, for example, we wanted to encourage a baby who was posterior or breech to turn. Putting in these front moves of the

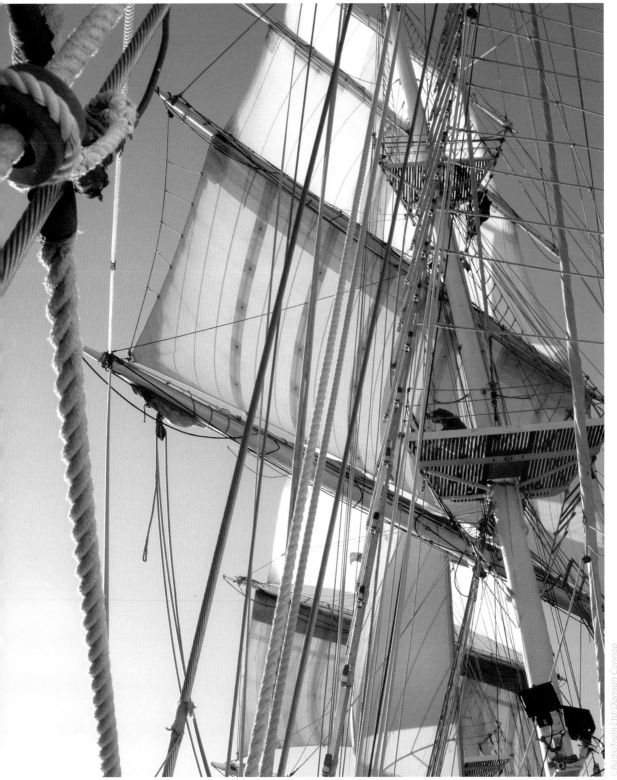

lower respiratory procedure helps to contain the impulses created by performing the pelvic procedure and greatly amplifies its effect in that area.

It is significant that in Bowen we perform moves on the front and the back fascia separately as there is a clear delineation which probably has its origins in our amphibian ancestors. We still have 'fishy' elements in our make-up that are remnants of this ancestory. For example, our hyoid bone is actually a remnant of a primitive gill.

In terms of evolution, we share with amphibians the separation of the viscero-cranium (the face, mouth, lungs and gut) and the neuro-cranium (the brain, spinal cord and vertebrae). Fascia is therefore structured in a similar way as having a clear delineation between the front and back of our body. Also in the embryo, the fascia that envelops organs arises from a different area of mesoderm to that of the structural bands of fascia.

Front and back fascia in humans have very different functions and dynamics which relate to our evolution not only from amphibians but also from being four-legged creatures.

Thus the back fascia (identified as the superficial back line by Thomas Myers) has a basic dynamic of tethering the body in an upright posture – a bit like the rigging on a ship. Without this we would fall forward. If you can imagine the back fascia on a four-legged animal going from four legs to two you will get the idea of the stresses involved.

In an animal, the front fascia supports all the abdominal organs as they hang down below the spine. In the neck, tubes of fascia hang down from the base of the cranium, particularly the sphenoid bone. In a human, a similar dynamic is taking place except that now in an upright position the fascia hangs down vertically. If we look at how the collagen fibres orient in the front fascia we will see it is very different front and back because of the very different stress factors put upon them. Again this can be related to the rigging on a ship (see image left).

It also explains the effect of 'holding points' in our work which will inhibit impulses travelling along these lines of fascia and contain and amplify these impulses in certain areas of the body.

Working with Scar Tissue

Because scar tissue can cause restrictions through the tissue field (not only structurally but also in terms of communication), it is sometimes very useful to work directly with it. Scar tissue responds very well to Bowen.

There are several ways of working with scar tissue. With recent scars it is better to work around the area rather than directly over it unless you can do surrogate work. With scar tissue that has settled you can do gentle moves directly over the scar. Tom Bowen used to work in this way by initially moving either end of the scar tissue and sometimes across the middle of the scar like this:

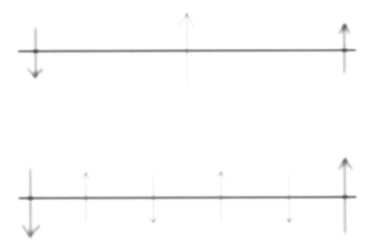

Research has shown that collagen fibres will re-orient themselves in response to the directional charge that is created by these types of move. This is probably why scar tissue responds so well to Bowen work and frequently becomes markedly less visible after a treatment. Some practitioners have also found that using some homeopathic remedies can help reduce scar tissue.

Dan Amato, a senior Bowen instructor in the USA, has postulated that the release created by a Bowen move creates a type of wave through the body called a soliton, the most well known example being a tsunami.

Solitons have interesting properties in that they carry large amounts of energy through the medium of water over long distances without loss. Interestingly, they also do not need a lot of pressure to set them off. The tsunami that devastated so many areas around the Indian Ocean on that fateful Boxing Day was actually set off by two tectonic plates colliding at the speed that our nails grow. In other words, it does not necessarily need a strong Bowen move to set up a strong response in the body. What is needed is enough pressure so that the body does not resist and therefore inhibit the response.

The effect of Bowen work on the fluidic elements of our bodies is highly significant. After all, we are at least 75% fluid. Loren Eiseley, the American poet whose work was so loved by the early cranial osteopaths, even described humans as being walking sacks of seawater – a not unscientific observation. In 1946 he wrote:

"Not for nothing has the composition of mammalian blood led to our description as 'walking sacks of seawater'. Not for nothing did the great French physiologist Bernard comment that 'the stability of the interior environment is the condition of free life.' The drifting cell masses of the early ocean lived in a nutrient solution. Salt and sun and moisture were accessible without great mechanical elaboration. It was the reaching out that changed this pattern, the reaching out that forced the cells to bring the sea ashore with them, to elaborate in their own bodies the very miniature of that all-embracing sea from which they came. It was the reaching out, that magnificent and age long groping that only life – blindly and persistently among stones and the indifference of the entire inanimate universe – can continue to endure and prolong."

Loren Eiseley, The Immense Journey, Vintage Books USA 1946

In his book *Job's Body*, Deane Juhan describes how easy it is for the fluid nature of our tissues, particularly what is called ground substance, to become stuck (he calls it fixotrophic) in response to accidents, falls and operations. It is as though the fluids become 'frozen' or more crystalline in nature and lose their ability to be responsive and malleable.

Bowen moves seem to unfreeze areas of tissue that have become frozen - Tom Bowen described it as 'freeing blocked energy' - possibly as a result of the strong energetic effect that Dan Amato describes.

Chapter 3

Embryological Development and the Uprising Midline

When Bowen therapists talk about a treatment allowing the body to re-orient to an original 'blueprint' or an organising principle, the question might be asked – what exactly is the body trying to orient to and when and how did this original blueprint arise?

The study of both cranial osteopathy and embryology might give us some clues.

As mentioned previously, osteopaths have written for many years how the forces that moulded the development of the embryo continue to express themselves right throughout life and if the practitioner can tune in to them, it allows the body to begin to re-organise itself to those forces.

James Jealous, an osteopath teaching in the USA, wrote recently:

"The Original design and function is in the fluids of the embryo... The Original matrix is a form that is carried through the potency of the breath of life around which the molecular and cellular world will organise itself into the Original pattern set forth by the Master Mechanic."

This might need some explanation. What Jealous is talking about is an organising force that is held in the fluids of the embryo – not necessarily just in the genetics. Interestingly, a number of eminent embryologists, including Bleschmidt and Jaap van der Wal, have questioned current thinking about the role of genetics in determining our structural and psychological make-up.

There is a lot of evidence to suggest that there is an organising force that goes beyond genetics and in fact arises epigenetically – some osteopaths think around the moment of conception or shortly after.

If one looks carefully at the first few days of embryological development, one notices that some very interesting events occur. At the moment of conception, there is a merging of the mother and father's DNA to form a single cell. After a moment of calm, there then occurs rapid cell division which happens within the outer 'shell' of the embryo, the zona pellucida.

Around day 15, a highly significant event occurs. A primal midline is established in the form of a furrow in the developing embryo. This primal midline is called the 'primitive streak' and it starts its uprising journey towards our embryonic heart at around the level that is later to become the coccyx and sacrum in the adult.

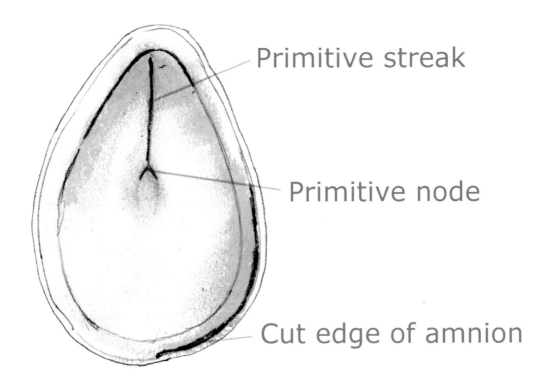

Primitive streak

Primitive node

Cut edge of amnion

The formation of the Primitive Streak around day 15

Why is this important? Firstly, the midline would appear to arise from something outside of natural cell division. What exactly initiates it is something of a mystery, but it forms the basis around which the whole body organises itself. Jaap van der Wal calls the emergence of the primitive streak, the 'finger of God'. If one sees a movie of this the nearest thing it looks like is someone drawing a line or furrow in the sand with a finger.

For a start it establishes a reference line for front/back, left/right and top/bottom. The primitive streak is referred to as an 'embryonic organiser' because it establishes a basic 'body plan'. Different levels of the primitive streak determine the development of different areas of the body. For example, the 'head centre' goes on to form the heart, brain and eyes, the middle centre the gut and trunk and the tail centre the pelvic organs and the neural tube.

In terms of left and right it determines, for example, the fact that the liver is on the right and the stomach on the left and the fact that the apex of the heart points to the left.

The primitive streak is something of a mystery to embryologists - it has been discovered that grafting of the primitive streak can cause an entire secondary axis to from around which cells will organise.

What is interesting for us as Bowen therapists is the importance of the primitive streak in terms of developing bones, muscles, organs and connective tissue. What happens is that as it emerges, it generates three definitive germ layers from the epiblast – endoderm, mesoderm and ectoderm. The mesoderm goes on to form somites at around day 20 when they first appear either side of the midline. These somites then go on to form the vertebrae and the limb buds of the arms and the legs.

Many Bowen therapists have remarked on the power of the first two Bowen moves to awaken a 'tissue memory' of health

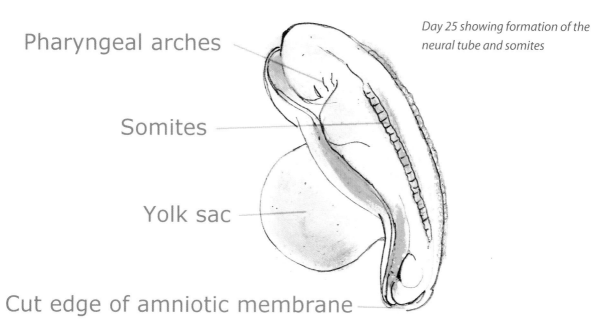

Pharyngeal arches

Somites

Yolk sac

Cut edge of amniotic membrane

Day 25 showing formation of the neural tube and somites

in the body. It is interesting to observe the sensations that start arising in the client after just these two moves. Many will have sensations of heat or an uprising force within the spine. In fact two Bowen instructors, Anne Schubert and Margaret Spicer, have constructed a whole new paradigm for Bowen they call 'mind-body Bowen' based on these moves alone.

The fact that so many clients experience an uprising force is interesting as their sensations correspond exactly to embryonic development as if those embryological forces were still present within the adult body. In Craniosacral therapy it is quite possible to palpate this uprising force by tuning into the notochord, whose remnants still exist in the centre of the inter-vertebral discs, and the apical ligament that connects the axis with the occiput.

In embryological terms what happens is that after the emergence of the primitive streak the midline it creates enfolds in on itself (literally bowing to the heart) to form the neural tube which then goes on to form the brain, spinal cord, the autonomic nervous systems (sympathetic and parasympathetic) and the neural crest.

Neural crest cells are very interesting as they migrate to various areas of the body during the development of the embryo. For example, they help form the inner membranes surrounding the brain and spinal cord (particularly the pia and arachnoid membranes, as well as myelin sheaths of nerves). In the coccyx procedure we move directly over the dura, arachnoid and pia

Transverse section of embryo showing development of neural tube during the fourth week

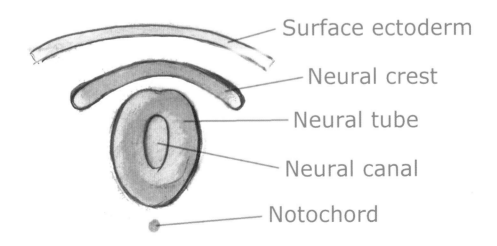

Surface ectoderm

Neural crest

Neural tube

Neural canal

Notochord

membranes as they attach to the coccyx in the form of the filament terminalis – the only place in the body where all the three layers of membrane come together.

Because of the coming together of these three layers of dura, arachnoid and pia, a very powerful impulse is sent up the spine towards the cranium (see chapter 10 on the coccyx).

Embryological development of tissue is very important in terms

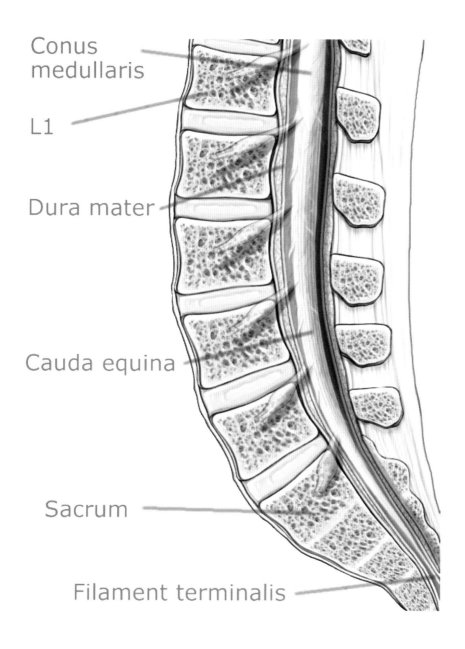

Conus medullaris

L1

Dura mater

Cauda equina

Sacrum

Filament terminalis

of referred pain. 'Head' zones are well known phenomena where, for example, someone might experience pain in their right shoulder as a result of a problem with their gall bladder. This is as a direct result of the embryology of the development of mesoderm, endoderm and ectoderm.

Another consequence of embryological development is the fact that blood supply and nerve supply to tissue is inextricably linked because of their derivation from the same embryological tissue.

Both L4 and C7 are also both highly significant in terms of the legs and arms in that these levels of the spine are where the buds which form the legs and arms grow out of. These levels are sometimes referred to as axial midlines.

When we talk about accessing a tissue memory of deep embryological organising forces, we are talking about cellular memory, particularly in the fluids and the liquid crystalline connective tissue of collagen fibres. The embryological development of collagen fibres is fascinating as it starts in the mesoderm (the middle layer between the ectoderm and endoderm) as fibrils, differentiates out to form different kinds of connective tissue in the body and then infuses all the layers of ectoderm and mesoderm. In other words, it becomes intricate to tissue throughout the body. It is well researched by Mae Wan Ho and others that collagen holds memory and that it is highly adaptable at registering new experience.

Is it possible that by stimulating the fascia we are in some way allowing the body to access and re-orient to these deep ordering forces held in the collagen at a cellular level in the body? From clinical observation, something of this kind certainly seems to be happening.

.

Chapter 4

The Esoteric

The idea of an inherent healing intelligence in the body has been central to all healing traditions throughout the ages. This is sometimes perceived as a powerful uprising force based at the sacrum (from the same root as the word 'sacred'). We have seen how this can be related to the 'original matrix' and embryological organising forces arising from the sacrum and coccyx as a midline. The manifestation of this primal organising midline is still somewhat of a mystery amongst embryologists.

In western healing this natural healing intelligence is represented by the caduceus, the symbol of the British Medical Association, whilst in Christian traditions it is mentioned in the writings of many mystics, including St. Therese of Lisieux and Hildegard of Bingen, as a rather misunderstood but powerful force capable of deep inner transformation. In terms of healing on a deep level, it allows direct perception of one's connection to creation and the divine.

Sometimes referred to as 'kundalini', it has been central to nearly all healing and religious traditions from the year dot.

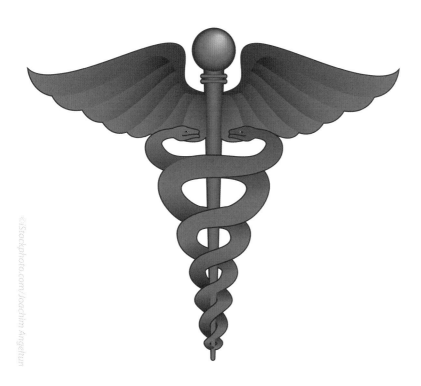

The Tibetan Buddhists refer to it as 'Cundali', where it is also known as the 'Yoga of the psychic heat' and is closely related to their practice of Tummo or the ability to generate inner heat (a useful tool in the cold climate of Tibet).

The interesting thing about kundalini though, is that the inner experiences are often similar across wide cultural boundaries: both Sufis and Hindus will report subtle movements in the spinal column followed by sensations of well-being and inner peace. As one member of the Kung people of the Kalahari who practise a trance-like dance to awaken the kundalini energy said:

"In your backbone you feel a pointed something, and it works its way up. Then the base of your spine is tingling, tingling, tingling, tingling, tingling, tingling...and then it makes your thoughts nothing in your head."

But what has this got to do with Bowen work? Although it is easy to make superficial similarities, there are some very interesting parallels. Kundalini awakening usually initiates an extremely powerful healing process in the body on many levels: physical, emotional, psychological and spiritual. This can sometimes leave the person quite confused (the many Kundalini sites on the web all carry 'government health warnings' about dabbling with this force unless you know exactly what you are doing). Certainly there are some alarming case histories reported of people who have undergone kundalini awakening 'by accident' as it were, and been through some horrendous times.

After working myself with kundalini for about 20 years it occurred to me that there must be a gentler, safer way of working with this kind of intelligent, healing energy. However, it wasn't until I came across both Bowen and Craniosacral work that I really felt I had found a way of encouraging someone's system to access this deep healing expression of 'the original matrix' in an entirely safe and structured way, albeit working from a slightly different perspective.

There is a lot written in sanskrit and vedic texts about the philosophy behind Kundalini. Traditionally, it is represented as a snake, curled up at the base of the spine, normally asleep. When awakened through various means like certain yogic practices, meditation, intense prayer, or just being around someone who has mastered their own state, the kundalini rises through the sushumna (the Brahma nadi or subtle nerve channel roughly corresponding to the centre of the spine), opening the various chakras as it rises until merging in the thousand petalled lotus at the crown of the head (the sahasrara).

This is under 'ideal' circumstances; in reality the path is not linear, and the person might experience the opening of various chakras in any order. In any case, the activation of these energy centres will bring with it an emotional, physical and spiritual response that can be very profound and very purifying on all levels. Most people will have experienced a similar opening of the heart chakra when falling in love.

The way the caduceus is represented shows two snakes intertwined around the sushumna. These represent the Ida and Pingala or the 'moon' and the 'sun'. They are also sometimes referred to as 'Ha' and 'Tha', from which we get the term Hatha Yoga. This practice was originally perceived to have a balancing effect on these two subtle nerve channels. Again, superficial parallels are not always useful, but there are some similarities here with the sympathetic nervous system and its plexuses. Some writers have also written on the parallels between the chakras and the endocrine system, although the subtleties of the different systems can get lost with comparisons like this.

On a 'cosmic' level the rising of the kundalini and its merging at the crown chakra represents a merging of Shiva and Shakti, or the transcendent and immanent, with Shakti being represented as the 'coiled feminine energy' at the sacrum and Shiva as 'pure consciousness' at the crown of the head.

Another way of looking at the rise of kundalini might be that huge reserves of intelligent, healing energy are released from their crystalline state at the sacrum (in yogic terms from the muladhara chakra at the level of the coccyx). As this energy is released, it helps to release patterns held within the tissues (tissue memory), opening up the system to an easier, more natural way of being.

In 'Devatma Shakti', the definitive Hindu treatise on Kundalini, this power is described as 'liquid light', which is also a term used by Dr. Sutherland, the founder of contemporary craniosacral osteopathy, to describe the 'Breath of Life' or the 'highest known element' – in other words consciousness itself. Some writers have also used the words 'liquid light' to describe the liquid crystalline nature of fascia.

Talking to many practitioners from many differing traditions, it is clear that the powerful healing properties of kundalini have close parallels in the expression of embryonic forces throughout life and a longing in the human being to get back to a primal state of health, well-being and connection with our true nature. Many clients report exactly this after a Bowen treatment - feelings of being at peace, a lifting of anxiety and connection to self.

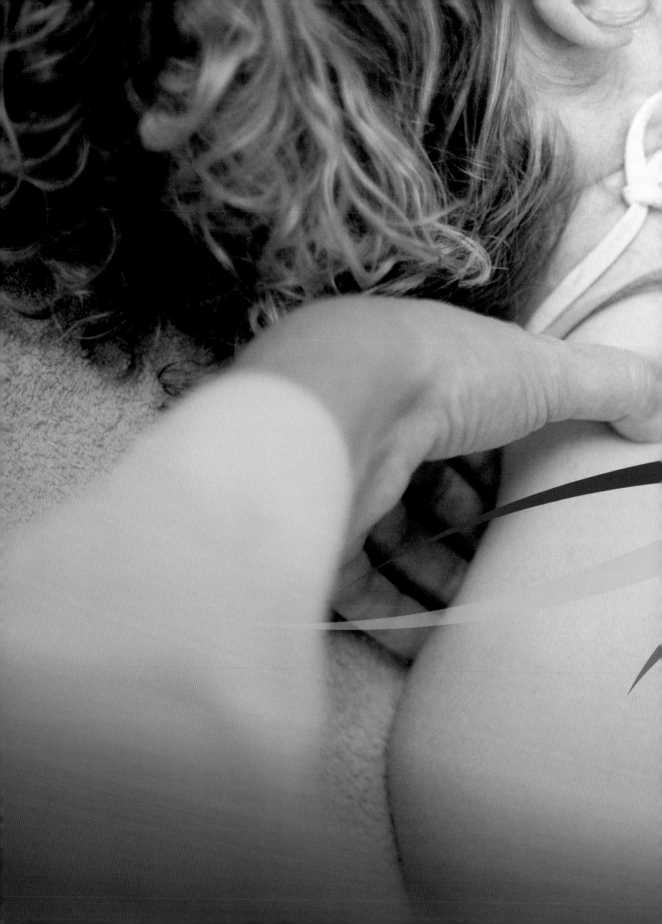

assessing the client

Chapter 5

Resources

How much to do?

The key to a successful Bowen treatment is in knowing how much to do. That is to say how many procedures or even how many moves within a particular procedure. As we know, Tom Bowen was a minimalist and with very good reason.

The closest analogy to Bowen work is homeopathy where the body is given a very small dose and asked to respond. If someone is half-dead, then there is not much point in giving it too much work to do – it simply can't do it, won't do it or will feel overloaded and overwhelmed. Either way, it is not helpful. In the same way, in a Bowen treatment we are giving the body small but targeted input so that it can begin its job of work to re-orient towards its original blueprint.

There are a few markers that will help us ascertain how much a person can take in terms of actual moves. I quite often take all these markers on a scale of 1 – 10 and do a rough tally in my head to determine how much to do with each client.

What we are looking for are the resources that they can bring to the treatment to assist them in recovery. These resources may be internal or external and can be classed as:

- Physical fitness
- Levels of toxicity in their system
- Emotional and psychological health
- Spiritual resources

Physical fitness really has nothing to do with how many times a week someone goes to the gym. It has much more to do with the quality of their muscle tone and the general level of fluidity in their body (see below).

This will also depend on how many operations or accidents they have had and/or what types of medication they may have taken. For example, cortisone injections which might be used to treat frozen shoulder or bursitis in the hip creates a lot of inertia and fixotrophia in the tissues and can therefore be much more time-consuming to treat.

Levels of toxicity will depend on their diet, use of drugs (recreational and prescribed) and whether they drink enough good quality water or not.

Homeopathy works on similar principles to Bowen when practitioners gauge what strength of potencies to give a client. George Vithoulkas writing in *The Science of Homeopathy* writes:

"There are certain types of cases in which relatively low potencies should be used – at least initially. The reason for this is that higher potencies can overstimulate weakened defense mechanisms, resulting in unnecessarily powerful aggravations [ie reactions]. This principle particularly applies to patients known to have specific pathology on the physical level – i.e., arteriosclerosis, cancer, coronary heart disease. When pathology has reached an advanced stage on the physical level, the constitution has likewise been relatively weakened, and administration of even the correct remedy in high potency can lead to severe sufferings. Thus in general it can be said that the more state of physical pathology, the lower the potency that should be used for the initial prescription."

The Science of Homeopathy, George Vithoulkas, Grove Press 1980

To the above list of patients with specific pathology I would also add anyone with autoimmune conditions (of which there are many different forms ranging from rheumatoid arthritis to lupus), chronic fatigue and ME, conditions that affect the central nervous system and peripheral nerves (Parkinson's, MS, Motor Neuron Disease etc) and severe imbalances of the endocrine system.

One way that Bowen differs considerably from Homeopathy is the occasionally perverse way reactions occur in differing individuals. This could be due to the fact that doing too much with clients or having too long a treatment session (and by too long I mean anything that involves them being on the couch for more than half an hour) can actually dampen the effect of the treatment.

Research in the USA has shown that that tissues respond better when there is a small amount of pressure on the connective tissue

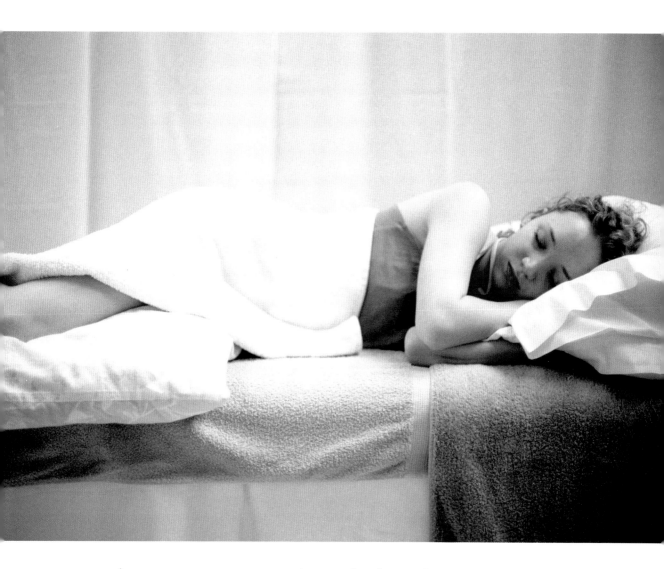

– too much pressure creates too strong a charge and makes repair less effective. Many physiotherapists have remarked that when they use ultrasound, it is often more effective to turn the machine to a lower intensity and treat for a shorter period of time. It has been estimated that the optimum impulse is at the level of nano-watts at around .75 milliwatt per square centimetre.

This is a very good case for 'the less is more' approach. However, it can lead to a confusing situation for a practitioner when they have to decide how much Bowen work to do with a client who is very unwell as a small amount of work can have such a powerful effect. One of the ways of playing safe with a client, especially on a first session when you may not be sure how they will respond, is to monitor their reactions closely during the treatment and leave longer gaps between moves.

For me Bowen is like a good tasty soup – the more you water it down the more insipid and unsatisfying it is. A very interesting (and not difficult) research project would be to measure the electrical impulses created by different pressures used amongst Bowen practitioners and see if there is any correlation between pressure and treatment outcomes.

Fluidity

One of the best ways off determining how someone will respond to the treatment and also how much to do with them is in terms of the natural fluidity of the tissues in their body, particularly muscles and fascia.

The efficacy of the treatment depends on impulses travelling along the lines of fascia, so if the fascia is dehydrated, cut (as in after an accident or operation) or fixotrophic (as Deane Juhan describes it), then impulses will not travel so well.

It is known that Bowen has a profound effect on fascia in terms of encouraging fluid into an area that was previously dry or inertial. This will change from treatment to treatment, but generally someone whose system is fluid will respond much more quickly to the work and will need less treatment, both in terms of number of sessions and also number of procedures or moves.

Hence, it is observed that babies and animals in particular need only minimal work to achieve profound change because their systems are generally so fluid and open.

Certain things will contribute to this. Drinking too much coffee, tea alcohol or sweet drinks will dehydrate the body. Hydration is controlled by the hypothalamus and the body will prioritise so that essential organs will remain hydrated. Connective tissue (including fascia and membranes) will be one of the first to dehydrate leading to adhesions and fixotrophia. If your client is suffering from a consistently dry mouth or other mucous membranes it is a sure sign that they are dangerously dehydrated. Similarly, headaches can be caused by dehydration of the membranes surrounding the brain and spinal cord which then tighten and put pressure on the nervous tissue. This is what happens in hangovers.

James Oschman in his excellent book *Energy Medicine* cites research which shows that a 10% increase in hydration (which is quite a lot when it comes to tissue hydration) will result in a million-fold increase in conduction of impulses through tissues such as collagen. This means our work could potentially be a whole lot more effective if we could get our clients more hydrated.

Some very interesting recent research has also shown that muscles will relax immediately when a client drinks water. This could be as a result of protons or electrons travelling almost instantaneously through the tissue fluid matrix. It would therefore be advisable to get clients to drink a glass of water (James Oschman suggests to add a small amount of salt to improve conductivity). Right before a treatment and when they get up from the couch. More details on this research can be found at www.energyresearch.bizland.com and in James Oschman's book *Energy Medicine in Therapeutics and Human Performance*.

Practices such as yoga and Pilates (particularly gentle stretching) encourage fluidity in the fascia and are an excellent complement to Bowen work. This is why people who practice yoga regularly usually respond so well to the treatment and need minimal input.

On the other hand, people who do fairly aggressive compressive exercises such as weight lifting or going to the gym regularly often damage the fascia through tearing. Muscles that are enlarged through such exercise is the result of tearing and bunching of the muscles fibres. This creates extreme lack of mobility in the fascia and a build up of toxins such as lactic acid and uric acid in the tissues. When such people are given a Bowen session for the first time they very often complain that they feel as stiff as a board for 24 hours after the first session.

Deane Juhan in his book *Job's Body* describes how the crystalline structure of fascia will be affected by under-use or over-use. Both

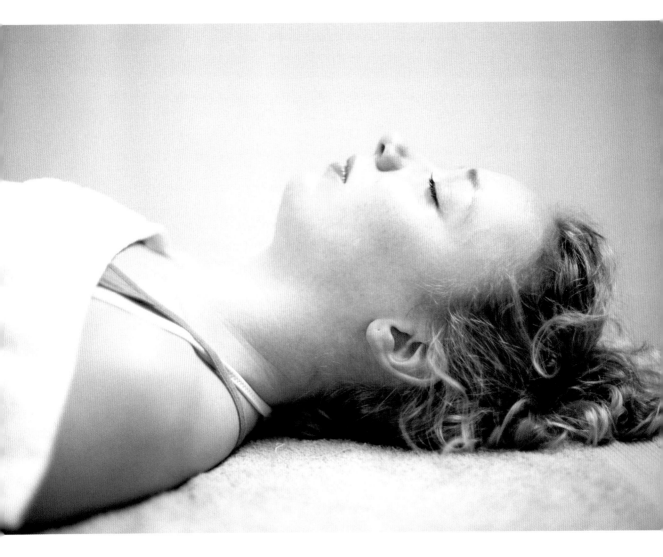

are undesirable in terms of Bowenwork. Hence, your average 'couch potato' who does very little in terms of exercise will have a lot of adhesions, density and toxins held in the muscles and fascia.

In my clinic, I have a good long corridor where I can observe people as they walk towards the treatment room. It is not difficult to see where someone is holding patterns of inertia as they walk. You will notice that certain areas of people's body will have more natural fluidity to them than others or they may have an 'awkwardness' in particular movements. These areas of lack of fluidity are often the areas one needs to work on fairly directly to change the fascial holding and drag in those areas.

Emotional and Psychological

In terms of fascia and other connective tissue, emotional armouring (as described by Wilhelm Reich, Stanley Keleman and others) can play a big part in people's receptivity to treatment.

For some people the intimacy of therapeutic touch can bring up all kinds of issues around vulnerability and can be experienced as quite threatening. It is essential for these people that we create a very safe environment in which to work and also that we find a way of accessing their system using our intention and light touch so that their bodies do not resist the treatment on a subtle level.

Negotiating resistance when giving a treatment is a fine art and needs a high degree of sensitivity. Sometimes, strangely enough, a firmer touch can feel safer for people who are not used to light-touch bodywork and can be a way in to allowing their systems to take on the work. Emotional armouring of this kind will be seen as rigidity in the tissues and is often there to protect the body against overwhelming experience.

When we realise that armouring often arises because of some strong or traumatic emotional event in the past, one realises that one must treat the person's system with a lot of respect. The protective pattern is there for a very good reason, even if that reason is no longer necessary and is quite possibly creating problems for the person. However, it could well be counter-productive to try and 'release' these held areas. It would be like taking away someone's walking stick and expecting them to walk effectively without it. They are likely to fall over and hurt themselves.

In the same way, traumatic held patterns in the body are often best negotiated from a distance, perhaps working around the area first for a few sessions before contacting the area directly.

Holistic and Spiritual Resources

One of the most positive aspects a client can bring to a session is an understanding of the holistic process and its part in their recovery. Someone who is used to taking allopathic medicine for a quick fix may not be too impressed if they have a reaction to a treatment for 24 hours.

A holistic understanding might include a need to change lifestyle or diet, an understanding that things might get worse for a short period of time before they get better and a commitment to drink plenty of water and exercise moderately.

It might also include an outlook on life that is intrinsically positive, for example that everything that happens can be used for personal growth, or that the universe is by its nature supportive and loving.

People with these positive aspects can take a little more work than someone who has a bleak outlook on life, who is depressed or maybe has just lost a loved one and is still grieving.

Feeling Good

For people who are in a lot of pain, either physical or emotional, it can be hard for them to find any place in their body that feels good and safe. It can therefore be very helpful, especially if they are having to deal with challenging situations in their life, to go through a simple settling exercise before starting treatment.

This involves them settling into some part of their body that feels good, warm and safe. In order for trauma to process effectively, there needs to be an awareness of present time and, most importantly, sensation in the body. Somatic Experiencing, developed by Peter Levine and described in his book *Waking the Tiger* and Babette Rothschild's work (see her books *The Body Remembers 1 & 2*), are both very useful in this regard.

Try these exercises with yourself before trying it with your client:

Settling Exercise

- Get yourself comfortable and in a place that is quiet, secure and where you will not be disturbed.

- If you are seated, make sure your feet are flat on the ground and that your back is supported on the back of the chair.

- Settle into your breathing, noticing the sensation of your ribs moving and the air entering and leaving your body. If you notice any tightness or restriction just acknowledge it without any attempt to change it.

- Bring your awareness to your feet and the sensation of contact of the bottom of your feet with the ground. Sink your awareness into the physical sensation of that without analysing or judging. As you move from the sensation of your left foot to the right, just notice the difference in feeling between the two.

- Try and hold the awareness of the plantar aspect of both feet together as they contact the floor.

- Move to the sensation of your buttocks on the chair. Sink into the physical sensation of that. Stay there for a while and notice how your mind begins to calm.

- Bring your attention to your arms and area of contact your forarms have with your lap. Rest your attention there for a few minutes.

- Moving back to your feet, see if it is possible to hold the awareness of the contact your feet have with the floor, the contact of your buttocks on the chair and the contact of your arms on your lap. See if you can hold all this in one unit of awareness. Stay there for a while.

- Now move to the sensation of contact that your back has with the back of the chair. Settle into that sensation.

- Again, go to your chest and the sensation of your chest rising and falling as you breathe in and out.

- Move your awareness to your face. Notice the sensations of all the muscles in your face. Are they tight? Are they relaxed? Without judgement and without wanting to change anything, just hold the physical sensation in your awareness.

- Lastly, see if it possible for your to hold all these areas of sensation in your awareness as one unit of awareness. Again, without judgement or wanting to change anything, settle here as long as you want to.

- When you are ready and before opening your eyes, very slowly bring your awareness out into the room, and if possible beyond. Settle there for a while.

- When you feel ready, slowly open your eyes and orient to your surroundings. Stretch and take a few good deep breaths.

Feeling Good Exercise

This exercise can be very useful for those suffering from traumatic overwhelm or who go into a situation during treatment where they get agitated, upset or are unable to settle. It can also be quite challenging for people who tend to identify with their suffering. It is a very effective tool for allowing such people to gain some distance and objectivity about their discomfort, whether physical or emotional. This exercise can also be given for clients to do themselves in the comfort of their own homes.

- Get into a comfortable position, either sitting or lying down. See if you can take a few minutes to settle into sensation – maybe the feeling of your chest as you breathe in and out or the feeling of your feet on the ground.

- When you are ready, get a sense of your body – does it feel easy or tense? Are there areas of your body which feel good and areas of your body that feel more difficult to feel comfortable in?

- See if there is an area that feels good, safe, warm and comfortable. This should be a physical sensation not just an idea. The place may be anywhere in your body – in your toe, thigh, pelvis, heart, throat or stomach. The important thing is that it can be felt as a physical sensation.

- If this is difficult, imagine a situation or activity you enjoy doing. This could be walking, swimming, lying on the beach etc. Imagine yourself being in this situation for a while. Go into the physical sensation of this – the warmth of the sun on your back or the feeling of waves lapping on your legs etc. See if you can stay with the physical sensation of that for a while and let it wash over you.

• As you do this, see if this pleasant sensation can spread out from this place into other areas of your body. If this is difficult, don't worry – just come back to your safe place.

• If this is enough for you, you can slowly bring yourself back into the room, open your eyes, stretch and orient to where you are.

• In further days when doing this exercise, you can see if you are able to begin to relate to areas in your body that feel less easy from this safe place. If you want you can 'shuttle' backwards and forwards from the safe place to the less comfortable place, or witness an uncomfortable place from your physical sensation for safety.

• When coming back into the room, do this slowly – give yourself plenty of time.

• If at any time during the exercise you feel yourself becoming frightened or overwhelmed, ask the question – what physical sensation tells me I am feeling fear/grief/anger etc.? It may be a tightness in the chest, a lump in the throat or whatever. Notice these sensations and see if they can just wave over you rather than you identifying with them. You can take some deep slow breaths and if things seem to be speeding up you can ask the question if these sensations would like to slow down.

This simple exercise can transform someone's relationship to their pain and allow healing to take place on a very deep level. When I was doing this exercise with some of the veterans of the war in El Salvador recently, they reported that it enabled them to get some distance from their psychological distress for the first time since the end of the war. For many people, their identification of themselves as something bad or guilty runs very deep and this simple exercise can be life-transforming.

If anyone has problems doing these exercises or become fearful during them, suggest they go and see a therapist who practises somatic experiencing.

Reactions

Tom Bowen used to consider a reaction where a client felt slightly under par for 24 – 48 hours after a treatment a good sign that the treatment was working. A reaction for longer than this would indicate that he had done too much.

What to do if someone has a reaction for more than 48 hours and is feeling uncomfortable?

This doesn't happen very often, but occasionally a client will forget to inform you that they have had a serious illness in the past. As the body moves towards health, the body will try and process latent illnesses. These may include old viral infections such as the herpes virus (round 80% of us carry the herpes virus in a latent form in our bodies) or autoimmune conditions such as lupus or rheumatoid arthritis.

Very occasionally if we have done too much with a client the body can react because it has become overwhelmed. This can be a difficult situation for both client and therapist as it is not necessarily a useful therapeutic process. The client may go into an inflammatory response where joints become more painful or conditions such as eczema re-surface for a while.

The best thing a therapist can do in this situation is maintain contact via the telephone, re-assure the client and suggest anti-inflammatory medication, homeopathy or herbal remedies, dependent on their areas of expertise.

If the client comes back in the following week still complaining of a worsening of symptoms, further extensive treatment is unadvisable as it will generally make the situation worse. However, performing the bottom stoppers, leaving the client for about 20 minutes, then doing the top stoppers and leaving them

for a further 10 minutes has been found by some practitioners to
be highly successful in alleviating a strong reaction.

Chapter 6

What goes up must come down (and vice versa)

Being an efficient Bowen therapist means being something of a Sherlock Holmes when it comes to ascertaining where the origins of someone's condition stems.

When it comes to structural or postural problems, one of the key things to establish is whether they are caused by ascending or descending influences in the body. This is not to say that both ascending and descending influences might not be happening at once. Unless one is treating someone who has minimal compensation patterns then usually both will be operating – although one or the other will usually be dominant.

Influences on how we hold ourselves come in all shapes and sizes – genetic, environmental, accidents, operations, emotional, spiritual and beyond.

However, if we are looking at a purely bio-mechanical or postural level (which of course will also influence and be influenced by emotional and other aspects) then the main ascending influences are:

1.   The plantar aspects of the feet (ie where the feet contact the ground)

2.   The ankles (particularly the lateral aspects)

3.   The knees

4.   The hip joints

5.   The pelvic floor

6.   The sacro-iliac joints

Conversely, the main descending influences (at least in terms of Bowen work) are usually:

1.   The temporo-mandibular joints (the TMJ)

2. The junction between the occiput and the atlas - sometimes called the 'rocker' (hence the expression 'off your rocker') or occipito-atlanteal joint (O/A junction)

3. The shoulders and thoracic inlet

4. The diaphragm

So, how to find out? Some simple markers might help.

Going Down

Firstly, descending influences on posture tend to start early in life (unless someone has had a whiplash injury or undergone extensive dental work).

It is often useful to ask the simple question – 'Do you remember as a teenager having a bad or 'weak' back. They will generally remember this more clearly as a teenager rather than as a child as the body goes through a series of growth spurts. If they say yes, then you need to look at working around these descending influences listed above, particulary the jaw.

The Jaw

Another way is to look carefully at their facial structures. I'm sure your mother told you never to stare at someone, but in this case you are excused. I have heard from many practitioners who knew Tom Bowen that he was very interested in facial markers, particularly the relationship between the eyes, the cheek bones (the zygomae and maxillae) and the jaw (the mandible).

To make this simple, imagine a horizontal line (or in some cases not so horizontal) going through the centre of the eye. Then imagine a similar line along the ridge of the cheek bones and also through the jaw. It will look something like *fig.1* right:

What we are interested in is the relationship between these three lines. Most dentists working in this field (and there are a few that work exclusively with the relationship between posture and bite, particularly in the child and adolescent) say that if there is a discrepancy in level between the jaw line and the cheek bones (and the other 2 are level), then the problem is likely to be coming from the bite (and particularly the TMJ). This might look something like *fig.2* right:

If, however, there is a difference in level between the cheek bones and the eyes (for example you may notice that one eye is narrower than the other), then the influence is likely to be more of a cranial one (particularly the relationship between the sphenoid (the bone that forms part of the socket of the eye) and the occiput. This will look something like *fig.3* right:

The possible reasons for facial asymmetry are numerous and do not necessarily concern us here. However, they may arise from birth patterns (particular types and positions of birth will tend to put different compressive forces on the baby's head – see the chapter on birth), or feeding patterns or later dental or orthodontic work.

Even though some of these patterns may have been established many moons ago in the life of our clients, it is still possible to work on them effectively. Compensation patterns, however long they have been going on for, are still held in the present time as highly energetic contained vortices, even if the need for that holding pattern arose a long time ago. However, because these patterns usually originated earlier in life it might be necessary to work on them over a longer period and not expect miracles overnight.

Osteopaths have remarked for many years on the similarity in construction between the TMJ's and the hips, and the pubis and the mandible and how they will tend to reflect each other in terms of compensation patterns.

An interesting side-line of our work could be in making our clients more eligible on the singles market – research has shown that people with facial symmetry are more likely to attract partners!

One of the major influences on the development of the hard palate and jaw is breast feeding. The strong suck of the baby on

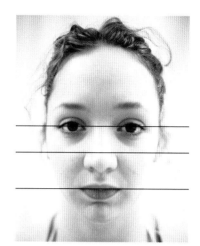

fig.1

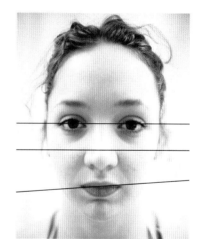

fig.2

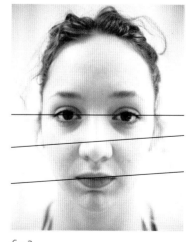

fig.3

the nipple helps mould the whole internal space of the mouth and hence will determine bite and dentition later on. A woman's nipple is perfectly designed to expand in 3 directions – side to side, top to bottom and front to back; not so an artificial teat, which unfortunately only expands in 2 directions (not front to back). The effects of bottle feeding (and also using a dummy) are therefore extreme in this regard alone, let alone the detrimental effect on the developing immune system.

The Neck

On one's case history form it is a good idea to include a question on whiplash injury. Many clients have suffered a minor or major car accident (though of course there are many other ways to sustain such an injury, particularly through horse-riding). Whiplash injuries tend to put a lot of strain on the upper cervical region, in particular the O/A junction. The muscles at the base of the occiput tend to be quite short and are therefore prone to damage, inflammation and atrophy after whiplash.

One tiny muscle, the rectus capitis posterior minor, is particularly vulnerable. It attaches onto the very base of the occiput beneath the trapezius and the semispinalis and goes down onto the

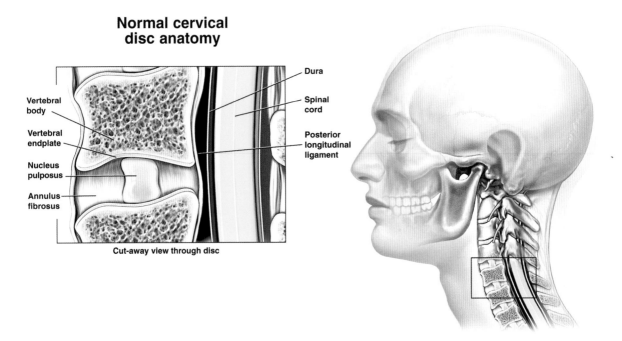

Normal cervical disc anatomy

Vertebral body

Vertebral endplate

Nucleus pulposus

Annulus fibrosus

Dura

Spinal cord

Posterior longitudinal ligament

Cut-away view through disc

transverse processes of the atlas. About 20 years ago during a dissection at an American dental college it was discovered that this little muscle had another important function. It was noticed that it also had attachments to the dural membrane that surrounds the spinal cord. It would appear that one function of this little muscle is to pull the dura out of the way when the neck is extended. Any atrophy of this muscle will inhibit this function, with resultant irritation of the dura.

You can feel this little muscle on yourself by placing your middle fingers just below your occipital crest and a finger's width below (where Bowen therapists perform moves 3 & 4 of the neck procedure). If you maintain gentle pressure here whilst just moving you eyes left and right you will notice a subtle movement of this muscle under your fingers.

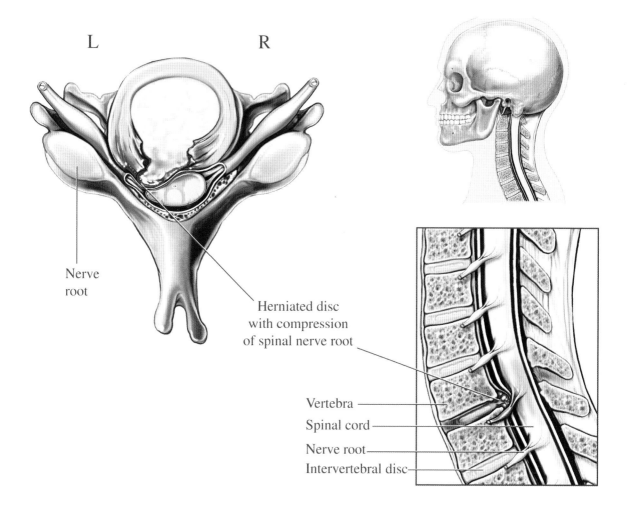

L   R

Nerve root

Herniated disc with compression of spinal nerve root

Vertebra
Spinal cord
Nerve root
Intervertebral disc

This instinctual movement is the remnants of a primitive head orienting response that develops in the womb and during the first years of life and it is mediated by nuclei in the brain stem.

Nerves are tender creatures and have particular adversity to being stretched or compressed (don't we all!). Sideways impacts can cause the nerves around the shoulder (the brachial plexus) to be suddenly stretched and compressed. The resulting damage and inflammation that sets in can then set off referred pain anywhere down the arm into the fingers. A study of the dermatomes will help ascertain which nerves are involved.

Shoulders

When one looks at the shoulder, you will notice that one is nearly always higher than the other – this usually depends on whether someone is left-handed or right-handed. The dominant hand (usually the right side) will be lower on that shoulder, which is quite normal. However, compensation patterns here may be related to a pelvic imbalance, TMJ issues or many other factors.

The Diaphragm

This dome-shaped muscle and tendon is hard to see and even harder to palpate but it is an important horizontal structure in its own right and will tend to influence and be influenced by everything above and below it. A lot of us hold all kinds of emotional and deep-seated angst in and around it.

Firstly, of course, there is the vulnerability of the solar plexus. The shock of having the umbilical cord cut too early (ie before it has stopped pulsating) can be a severe shock for the little one – a shock that can be held long into life – and is referred to by psychologists as umbilical effect (see chapter on birth).

A remnant of our umbilical vein forms our falciform ligament which goes right the way through our liver and it is common for umbilical shock to be fed directly into that area partly because some very rapid changes have to happen in the liver straight after birth.

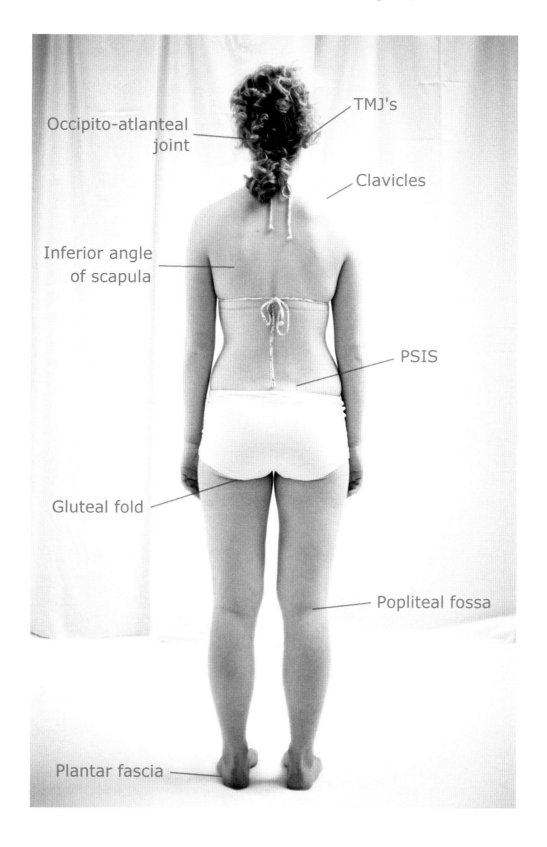

Occipito-atlanteal joint

TMJ's

Clavicles

Inferior angle of scapula

PSIS

Gluteal fold

Popliteal fossa

Plantar fascia

The diaphragm also has deep connections with the psoas major – a muscle which travels deep down and attaches on to the top of the femur at the lesser trochanter. This muscle can hold deep and primal feelings to do with survival and fear.

The area of the back where the posterior attachments of the diaphragm are (around T12) is incredibly important posturally, being a kind of fulcrum for the body in the relationship between the trapezius and the psoas.

Going up

In some ways, ascending influences are easier to observe than descending ones. The usual physical landmarks we use for assessment here are:

1. The medial malleolus

2. The crease at the back of the knee (the popliteal fossa)

3. The gluteal fold (horizontal crease at the base of the gluteus maximus)

4. The sacro-iliac joint (particularly the PSIS or the dimples at the back of the pelvic crest)

5. The iliac crests

There are several things one might observe here. Firstly, the horizontal levels of these landmarks; you may notice a difference in the level of the gluteal fold – this will usually tell you that there is some pelvic imbalance.

The 'dimples' at the PSIS can tell us a lot about the sacro-iliac joint – are the dimples level? Is one dimple more pronounced than the other? Is there 'puffiness' or an appearance like a hot water bottle around the sacrum beneath the dimples? This may indicate some inflammation around the sacrum and its ligaments.

As the client is standing, look at the angle of their feet – is one more turned out than the other? This may indicate a tightness

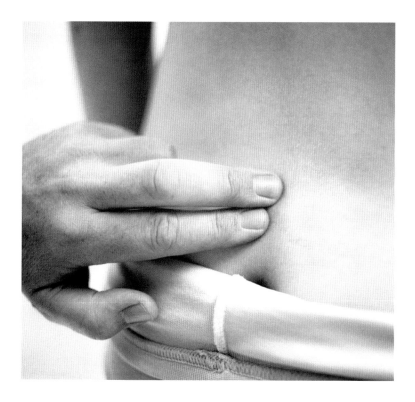

through the piriformis on the side that is more turned out (ending up in a duck-like gait). Where the leg has a tendency for being turned in towards the midline, this might indicate a tightness through the psoas or the adductors.

The Feet

The plantar aspects of the feet are the primary transverse relationship in the body. If anything is 'up' here it will reflect in every other transverse relationship.

So, what can go wrong? Well, we are looking at pulls through any part of the fascia of the foot as well as any hypermobility in any of the toe joints.

Supposing your client has a hypermobile big toe joint on their right foot. Every time their right leg hits the ground it will not be supported on the medial aspect. This will then create a pull up into the knee and from there into the hip, pelvis and sacro-iliac joints.

Supposing they have at some stage broken a bone in their foot.

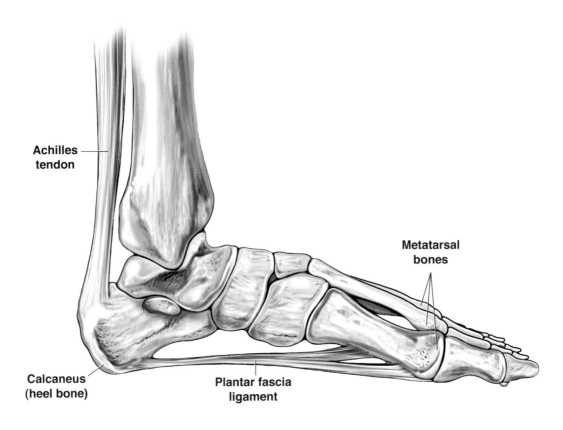

Achilles tendon

Metatarsal bones

Calcaneus (heel bone)

Plantar fascia ligament

Very likely the fascia around that area will be tight and will pull into the Achilles tendon and up into the gastrocnemious. Given the nature of fascia as liquid crystal this will affect the whole fascial 'train' from its beginning to end.

The Ankle

The most common ankle problem affects the lateral ligaments, particularly the anterior tibio-fibular ligament (ATFL). If this is a repeated injury in a clicnt it is likely to be a postural problem, possibly coming from their hip or pelvis which needs addressing. However, locally this can cause problems up the lateral aspect of the leg into the ilio-tibial band and into the hip.

Generally speaking the longer someone has had a condition the more the body will have to set up compensation patterns. From the therapist's point of view this means the more they will have to address the whole body rather than just locally as in an acute situation.

The Pelvis

In the next chapter we shall look at ways of assessing the body, particularly in relation to issues affecting the pelvis.

Chapter 7

Orthopaedic Tests

It is advisable to undertake any physical assessments, orthopaedic tests or palpation before beginning a treatment session so that we do not interrupt the flow and relaxation of the session. It is also very important to understand what precisely you are testing for and not to diagnose. We are merely using these tests to help us ascertain where we need to work and what procedures or what moves of a procedure will be most effective. Remember, if you only address the area of pain, then at least 70% of the time you will be working in the wrong place.

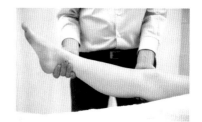

What tests we decide to use will depend on the presenting symptoms. However, for lower back issues, sciatica, femoral nerve pain and disc problems, the straight leg raise test and the sacro-iliac test both yield a bounty of information.

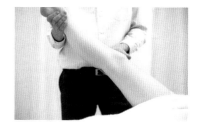

The Straight Leg Raise Test

This is so much more than it says on the can. This test involves simply raising the leg slowly, supporting under the back of the knee and the ankle with the client lying on her back. As the leg is raised passed about 35 degrees (try and get the client to relax the leg as much as possible and not assist), it begins to pull on the nerve roots and the dural sleeves that surround them in the sacrum and the lumbar area. As you raise up to about 80 degrees, the stress on the dura increases. After this point no further stress is created.

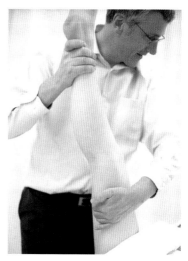

The first part of this test, therefore, is used to ascertain if there is any nerve entrapment where the nerve exits the foramina of the lumbar and sacral areas. This can be as a result of a prolapsed disc (though this will usually only show up with an acute disc problem where there is inflammation) or entrapment of the dural sleeve that encases the nerve as it exits the spine.

As you raise the leg anywhere between about 35 – 80 degrees, the client may feel an increase of pain, numbness, or tingling anywhere down the leg, in the foot, in the buttock, hip or back. Obviously, as soon as the client feels any of these symptoms we stop the test as we do not want to aggravate or inflame the condition.

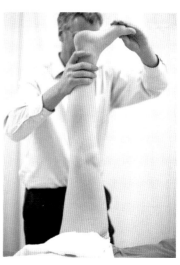

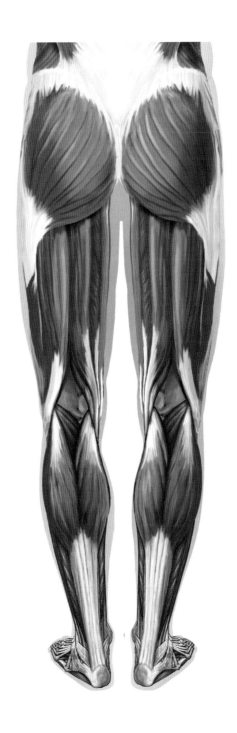

It is important to ask the client where exactly they feel the pain, numbness or tingling as this will tell us what nerve root is affected. If they feel it in their big toe, for example, it will be the nerve root at L4 or L5 that is affected. If it is the back of the knee, it will be S1 or S2; if it is the groin it will be the femoral nerve at around L2. It is fairly easy to trace the source of a nerve, so it is worth having charts to hand that show dermatomes, mytomes and scleratomes – these are the areas of skin, muscle and bone respectively that are innervated by particular nerves.

If this test is positive, what it tells us is that we need to work around the area of the back that is affected as that is where the nerve entrapment is happening, despite the fact that they may be feeling it in their foot or somewhere else. We also need to look at what postural or other issues may be causing this entrapment.

Because embryologically the same nerves form dermatomes, myotomes and scleratomes, it is possible for a client to say, for example, that they feel a pain or numbness in the front of the thigh, tightness in the adductors or psoas or pain deep in the hip. It is not unusual for clients to feel pain in different places (they will usually say it is deep in the muscle or deep in the bone or as sensitivity or numbness in the skin), even though that there is only one nerve involved. Charts can help track the origin of these sensations to where the nerves exit the spine.

The second part of the straight leg raise test involves seeing if there is any tightness or restriction in the myofascial tissue from the lumbar through to the plantar fascia of the foot.

As you raise the leg, assuming there is no increase in nerve sensation, you will at some stage begin to feel resistance. Without stressing the leg too much, you can ask the client exactly where they feel the restriction or tightness (as opposed to pain which is something else). It is important to get the client to be as precise as possible as they may be feeling the restriction anywhere from their lower back, hip, sacrum, hamstrings, knee, calf muscles or even into their feet. If they feel it anywhere down the leg, ask them whether it is more on the inside (medial) or outside (lateral).

This information will tell you exactly where you need to work and which procedure you need to do. For example, if they feel it more in the calf muscles (the gastrocs), then the knee procedure would be appropriate. If it is more in the sacrum, then the sacrum procedure rather than the hamstring work would be more suitable.

Now for a bit of fun. To demonstrate how effective Bowen moves are in freeing up restrictions in fascial tracts, try this exercise. First, perform the straight leg raise test. Notice the precise area of restriction (not pain) i.e. is it medial, lateral – an area in the gastrocs, behind the knee, in the hams, the sacrum, hip or lower back? Having isolated the area exactly, perform only one move right over the area of restriction. This might be any move from any of the procedures – for example move 4 of the hamstrings or move 8 of the knee etc. It is very likely you will find different areas of restriction on the right leg to the left leg. Allow the client to rest and pay particular attention to reactions that occur, being very careful not to interfere until reactions have settled down. Get the patient up to walk around for a minute and then re-test using the straight leg raise test.

It is not known if Tom Bowen worked in this way, but students have found this exercise a very powerful demonstration of the power of minimalist work.

The Sacro-iliac Test

In humans (and in horses that carry humans on their backs), the sacro-iliac joints are particularly prone to getting locked up, as described in the section on the Sacral procedure.

The sacro-iliac test really is a must if you want to ascertain whether or not you need to do the sacral procedure on a client. Typically, a client with a locked sacro-iliac joint will complain of sciatic pain (often radiating down to the foot), stiffness in the lumbar, and frequently a related neck restriction.

The test is performed with the client standing. Make sure that you have a suitably high backed chair or some other sturdy furniture so that the client can support themselves with one hand.

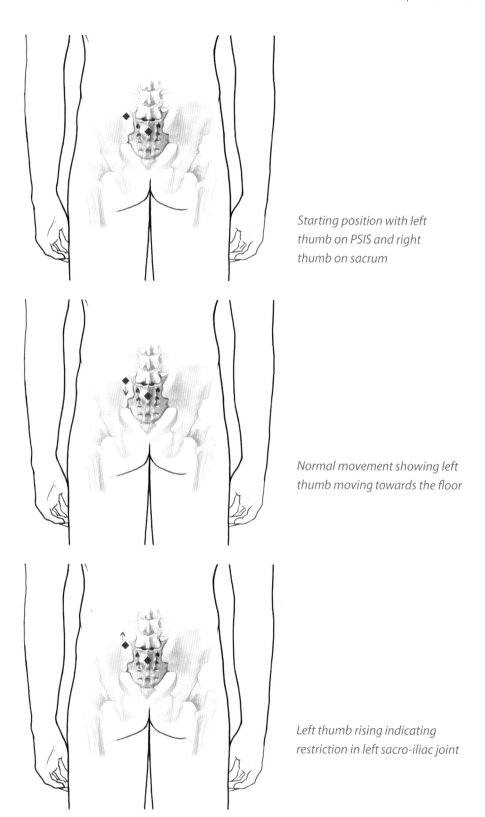

Starting position with left thumb on PSIS and right thumb on sacrum

Normal movement showing left thumb moving towards the floor

Left thumb rising indicating restriction in left sacro-iliac joint

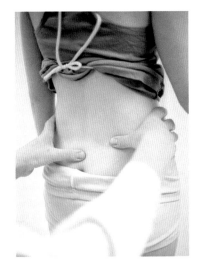

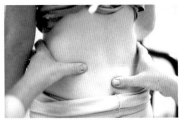

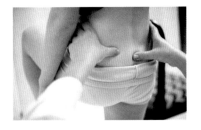

Firstly, identify the centre of the sacrum – this will be just above the top of the gluteal crease. Place the thumb of your right hand on the centre of the sacrum. With the thumb of your left hand, identify the left PSIS (posterior superior iliac spine). This will be just lateral to the dimples if they are visible. The other way of finding this point is to trace the line of the iliac crest posteriorly until you come to the PSIS. Rest your left thumb there. Ask the client to raise their left knee towards their chest. You will get a better reading if the client can raise the knee just above the 90 degree angle or, alternatively, until the thigh is above parallel with the ground.

In an ideal situation, the left PSIS should lower towards the floor significantly by about a good centimetre and a half. If it goes up or stays stationary, there is a restriction on that side. The degree to which it goes up or stays stationary gives an indication of the severity of the restriction. Change hands and do the same procedure on the right S/I joint.

With elderly, infirm clients or those where it is too painful to raise their knee, you can do the same test by simply asking them to step forward on their left and then right feet. The results of a lowering iliac crest are more difficult to see but straightforward with practice.

A positive result will indicate whether or not the sacral procedure is indicated.

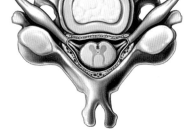

Cervical vertebra with spinal cord and intervertebral disc

The Slump Test

This test is used to ascertain whether there is any restriction in mobility of the dural sleeves surrounding the spinal nerve roots as they exit the spinal column. This kind of restriction is very common with symptoms of 'trapped' nerves or inflammation of neural tissue.

As each spinal nerve exits the spinal canal it is enclosed in a sleeve of dura, rather like the arm is enclosed in the sleeves of a short-sleeved shirt. Freedom of movement of the dura is essential as the body bends and twists during the normal course of events in the day.

Restrictions are commonly caused by vertebral subluxation but can also be affected by restrictions in the sacro-iliac joints and in the neck. What tends to happen is that restrictions pull on the dura causing irritation and inflammation in the nerve tissue. When neural tissue becomes inflamed it swells, and this creates a vicious cycle of nerve activation.

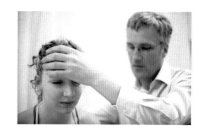

The slump test involves the patient sitting on the edge of the couch with the knees fairly well forward. It is a good idea if the practitioner sits or stands next to the client so that you can support the client's body and stop them falling. This test needs to be done very slowly for safety's sake. It is very important to stop the test as soon as any pain or discomfort is felt.

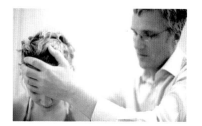

The first part of the test involves the patient bringing their head slowly down towards their chest. It is a good idea if the practitioner supports the client's head in this process by putting one hand on the forehead and the other on the occiput. Remember to stop as soon as any pain is felt.

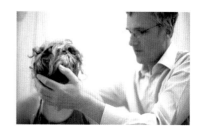

Assuming there is no discomfort, the next part involves the patient's whole body 'slumping' forwards, again with the practitioner supporting at the forehead and occiput. The last part is asking the client to slowly straighten one leg with the foot in dorsiflexion.

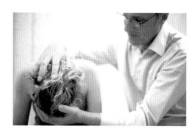

We need to be clear that we are testing for any activation of nerves as a result of the test. We are not in this instance looking for restriction. What this test does is stress the whole dural membrane (what Dr Sutherland called the reciprocal tension membrane) from the coccyx through to the cranium. It therefore shows up any areas where the dura is restricted and causing pressure on the nerve. For this reason the client may feel the pain or discomfort in any area supplied by a particular nerve – for example, they may feel discomfort or tingling in the arm as a result of restriction of the nerve roots in the neck. We have to be something of a detective in tracing the source of the pain back to a particular area of the back, but what a positive response to this test shows us is that we need to specifically work the area of the back where the restriction is occurring. This may need some explanation to a client if you are working on their lower back for a pain they feel in their knee, for example.

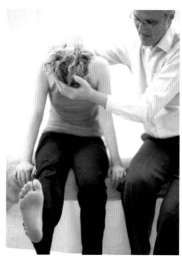

The brachial plexus

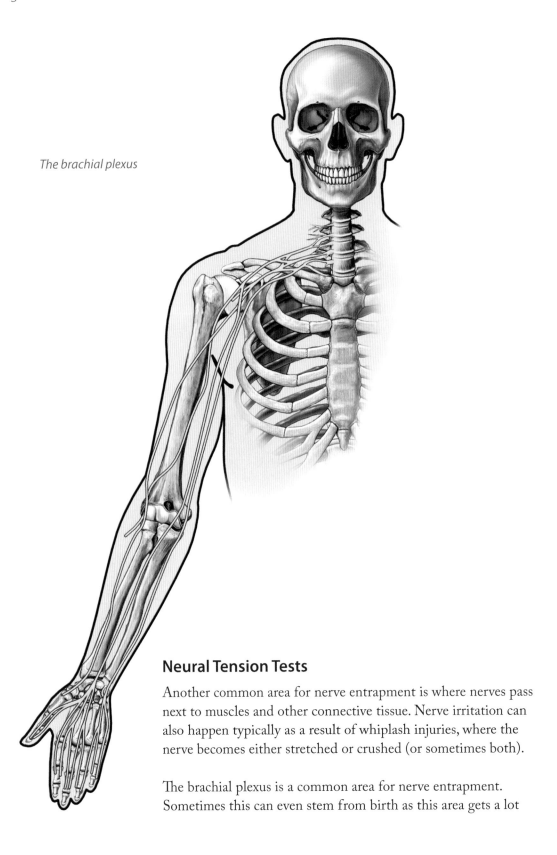

Neural Tension Tests

Another common area for nerve entrapment is where nerves pass next to muscles and other connective tissue. Nerve irritation can also happen typically as a result of whiplash injuries, where the nerve becomes either stretched or crushed (or sometimes both).

The brachial plexus is a common area for nerve entrapment. Sometimes this can even stem from birth as this area gets a lot

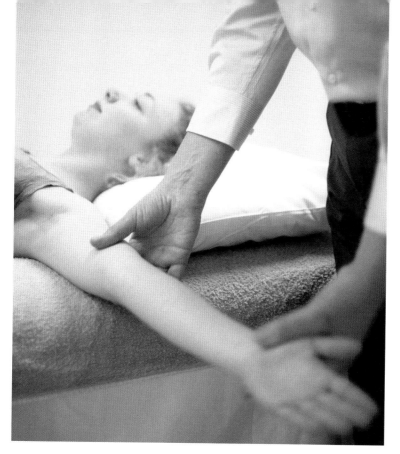

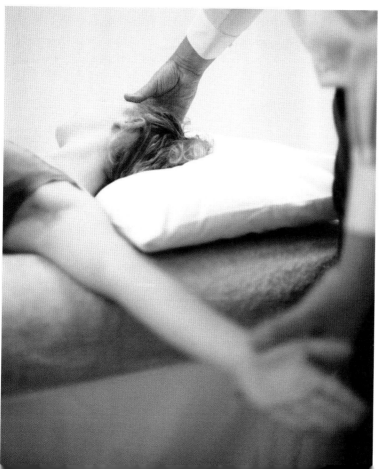

of stress during the birth process depending on which shoulder is born first in a normal vaginal delivery. If nature is left to run its course, the posterior shoulder will naturally emerge first. However, in a lot of hospital deliveries the anterior shoulder will be encouraged out first and this puts a lot of stress on this side (normally the baby's right shoulder).

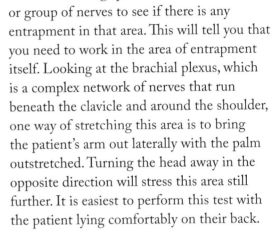

Neural tension tests involve stressing specific areas of a nerve or group of nerves to see if there is any entrapment in that area. This will tell you that you need to work in the area of entrapment itself. Looking at the brachial plexus, which is a complex network of nerves that run beneath the clavicle and around the shoulder, one way of stretching this area is to bring the patient's arm out laterally with the palm outstretched. Turning the head away in the opposite direction will stress this area still further. It is easiest to perform this test with the patient lying comfortably on their back.

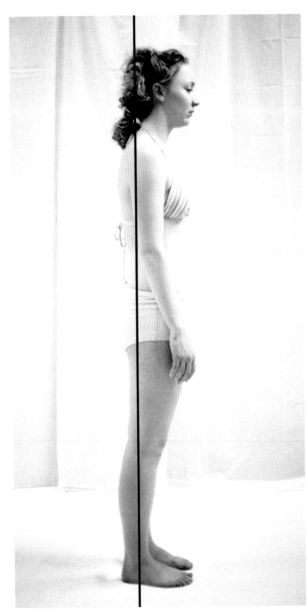

Bowen procedures that address the brachial plexus area specifically are the chest, east, non-response and levator trapezius procedures. Usually only one of these procedures on one side of the body is sufficient to address the problem.

Some practitioners use a 'plumb line' to assess postural anomalies. It is fairly easy to do this and can give a lot of useful information. If the client stands behind the line, get it aligned with their lateral malleolous with their feet comfortably spaced but at the same level. Notice what structures the plumb line passes through. It should ideally bisect the hip joint (this will be just posterior to the great trochanter), the shoulder capsule and the ear canal (the TMJ). If you assess the client both left and right it will be easy to see any rotational patterns they are holding through their spine; for example, their shoulder might be more anterior or posterior on one side.

Most people in the west have an anterior head position (head forward posture), which will result in an anterior pelvis and hip. The head is very heavy and so holding this anterior position throughout life puts a huge strain on the back, particularly the lower lumbar area.

One can also observe how someone is standing in terms of the angle of their feet and which areas of the heels of their shoes are most worn.

A normal angle of the feet when they are standing, or lying down on their back (called the Fick angle) is where the feet have a slight tendency to rotate outwards. Where there is excessive rotation outwards on one leg it might indicate a tightness in the piriformis muscle on that side resulting in a 'duck-like' gait.

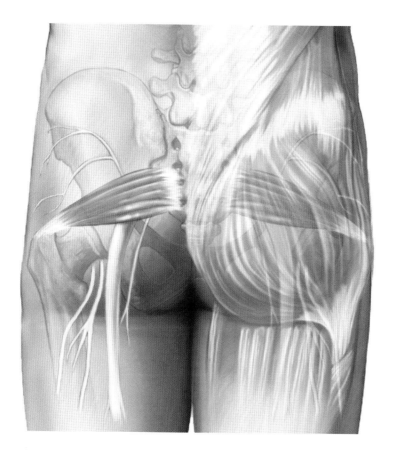

The piriformis muscle and sciatic nerve

Physiotherapists often give specific exercises to relax this muscle, such as encouraging the patient to walk with their toes pointing more to the front. However, in Bowen work, we prefer to allow the body to adjust of its own accord without interference. Tightness in the piriformis muscle might affect the sciatic nerve causing irritation and sciatica or leading to a vicious cycle of muscle spasming. One of the best ways of addressing this area is to perform the 'buttock pain' procedure. This involves doing the coccyx move from the side of the painful piriformis, waiting 20 minutes and then doing the other side of the coccyx and leaving the client for 10 minutes. This can be a powerful way of addressing piriformis pain as well as sciatic pain in general, even when it radiates down the leg.

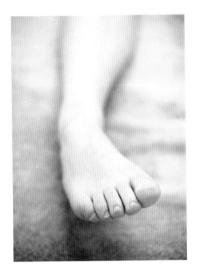

Observations

Much can be observed with the client lying on their back, however it is important to realise that what you observe with the client lying down may be very different when they are standing up.

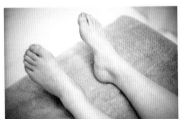

It is worth looking at the angle between the lower part of the leg (the tibia and fibula) and the foot.

Where there is an angle at the ankle as in the illustration, it will usually indicate a pelvic or hip issue. This sort of position will also put a lot of strain on the knee and it is likely they will have a tendency to injuries there.

It is also straightforward to see any imbalance in the pelvis by placing your thumbs just below the medial malleolus, bringing the legs together and seeing if your thumbs are level. I usually get the client to first lift their pelvis whilst their knees are bent and then apply some gentle traction on the legs after they have lowered their pelvis. This tends to give a better reading because unless the legs are straight it is easy to get a false reading.

Orthotics

The issue of whether orthotics can help or hinder the effects of a Bowen treatment is a controversial one. It seems in any case advisable to ask your client to refrain from wearing them during the few days after the treatment to allow the body to adjust. I have treated many clients in the past with apparent leg length discrepancy who have been told they needed to wear orthotics. Mostly after a series of treatments they are able to do without. Looking at possible issues with the feet is important, especially when posturally-related symptoms return. One alternative to orthotics is the use of the foot strengthening system developed by *Barefoot Science* which consists of insoles along with a number of progressive strengthening inserts. Jonathon Damonte, a senior instructor in Vancouver, has used these effectively for many years, particularly in cases where Bowen work doesn't 'hold'.

Chapter 8

Working with Chronic Pain and Facilitation

Inflammation
may turn out to be
the elusive Holy Grail of medicine—
the single phenomenon
that holds the key
to sickness and health.

J Meggs, MD The Inflammation Cure

Chronic pain presents a real challenge to a Bowen therapist, as it is often so difficult to ascertain the origin. By chronic pain, we are talking about a situation that has persisted for more than six weeks.

Part of the problem is that the longer pain persists, the more scope there is for referred pain, for compensation patterns to be set up, and that it will spread and become more entrenched. Where there is a level of inflammation in the tissues, which is nearly always the case, chronic pain will affect not only the peripheral nerves and the spinal cord, making them hypersensitive, but it will also have an activating effect on the sympathetic nervous system.

The sort of situations or conditions that might create this scenario are:

- Any inflammatory condition

- An injury to a joint (knee, ankle, wrist, shoulder, elbow etc) that has not completely healed

- Adhesions (eg around the ovaries or after operations)

- Fibroids

- Vertebral subluxations that put strain on the ligaments and muscles around the spine

- Root canal fillings

- 'Slipped discs' where there is inflammation

- Scar tissue, particularly where it is still mildly sensitive

- Any tissue damage that has not healed or there is still mild aggravation

If it is chronic, it is usually easy enough to spot someone who is suffering from this because they will be exhibiting all the symptoms of an over-active sympathetic system:

- An inability to sleep well

- Anxiety (could be low level) or panic attacks

- Raised blood pressure or palpitations

- Potential loss of appetite

- A tendency to become quickly emotional or angry

- A change in skin tone and texture around the site of injury (for example the skin may become thinner and drier)

One of the most crucial things I have found is to try and address this activation of the sympathetic nervous system first before anything else. It is a physiological fact that it is very difficult for the body to repair unless the parasympathetic – sympathetic balance in the body is restored. In any case, once the activation of the sympathetic system becomes lowered, they will begin to feel so much better in themselves.

Ways of addressing the SNS are primarily via the BRM's moves 9 – 16, the kidney (because it addresses the adrenals), the coccyx (because of the sympathetic and parasympathetic nerves in that area) and the TMJ (because it stimulates the Vagus nerve, the major parasympathetic nerve in the body).

It may take a few treatments for the system to begin to settle and one would not do all of the above procedures in a single session. Best to go slow, leave long gaps and KISS (keep it simple, stupid!).

Once the system has settled (and you will know because the patient will feel and look much better in herself and the perception of pain will have lessened), then you can go on to address the area of the original pain, whether it be an arthritic hip, a broken wrist that hasn't healed properly or a slipped disc etc. It is also a good idea to address the area around the spine that is affected by performing any appropriate lateral moves (for example the kidney, moves 9 – 16 or the lower respiratory). These can have the effect of dissipating some of the high electrical charge held there. The kidney procedure is particularly useful for any chronic pain affecting the lower back because it addresses the area of the spinal cord where so much of the nerve impulses are processed.

Osteopaths have a term for when the nervous system becomes sensitised and the spinal cord is affected. They call it facilitation, or in the case of the spinal cord, a facilitated segment, which is a level of the spinal cord that has become hypersensitive. The word facilitation refers to the fact that nerve impulses travel along the nerves and are created much more easily than they should.

What happens is this:

As a result of chronic inflammation, nociceptors, which are small, high threshold sensory nerve fibres that sense tissue damage begin to break down and become hypersensitive. This can happen as the result of any kind of on-going inflammatory condition, for example endometriosis, inflammatory bowel disease, IBS, tissue damage in a knee or ankle, an arthritic hip, an old operation scar, inflammation around adhesions or inflammation in the vertebral ligaments or the inter-vertebral discs themselves (particularly around the posterior part of the disc which is high in nociceptors).

One reason why it is so difficult to ascertain the source of chronic pain is because there are so many possibilities as to the origin, and frequently there is more than one source operating at once. When one hurts oneself and there is some tissue damage of some kind, there is a natural release of various neuro-active substances which are designed to work well on a short-term basis. Substances such as endorphins, histamines, prostaglandins, adrenaline and cytokines are all released to aid tissue repair in a co-ordinated onslaught.

The thing to understand is that one can get sensitivity created because of inflammation in an organ (for example a kidney infection or a condition such as endometriosis) that then affects the muscles which are controlled by the same spinal segment. One can also get the reverse happening where some tissue damage in a joint or muscles can affect organs at the same level.

What you will notice is that the area of the spinal cord that is affected (particularly around the erector spinae muscles) will display the following characteristics:

- The skin will be drier or rougher at that level (in some cases there will be tufts of hair around it, or the skin will have an 'orange peel' texture).

- The erector spinae muscles will be both hard and sensitive locally. For example, you may be working up the back and come to an area where the muscle suddenly 'jumps' and is sensitive.

- There will be an energetic 'buzziness' to the area of the spinal cord. If you gently bring your hand up or down the spine around an inch from the body, you may have a sensation like you are close to a high voltage electricity line at some point. This sensation is slightly different to other feelings that one might palpate in other parts of the body. Heat, for example, might be due to inflammation or (if you are a healer or Reiki practitioner) might indicate that the body is drawing 'healing energy' in that area. Coldness, or a cold streaming as though someone is blowing on your hand, can often indicate that an area of the body has been exposed to some physical impact. Dr John Upledger calls this phenomenon a 'force vector'.

- Redness or whiteness will appear on the skin which will last a good few minutes. Redness which comes and goes fairly quickly is not so significant and some people can be naturally sensitive to the acidity in one's hands. Sometimes one might also notice a red 'streaming' on the skin which follows the path of a spinal nerve. Redness like this is a result of the cells releasing histamine – an activity mediated by the Sympathetic Nervous System.

- The spinous processes may be sensitive at that area. A gentle tapping may result in a subtle contraction or 'jumping' of the muscles around the spine.

It is very useful to be able to track where the nerve irritation and hence original tissue damage and inflammation might be coming from, bearing in mind that the origin might be somatic (tissue, joint etc) or visceral (organ), and also what areas of the body (again somatic or visceral) this nerve facilitation might be affecting.

Complex Regional Pain Syndrome

One classic example of this is what is now termed Complex Regional Pain Syndrome (CRPS). CRPS used to be referred to as "reflex sympathetic dystrophy syndrome" and "causalgia," a term first used during the American Civil War to describe the intense, hot pain felt by some veterans long after their wounds had healed.

The key symptom of CRPS is continuous, intense pain out of proportion to the severity of the injury or tissue damage, which gets worse rather than better over time.

According to the National Institute of Neurological Disorders in the USA, CRPS most often affects one of the extremities (arms, legs, hands or feet) and is also often accompanied by:

- burning pain

- increased skin sensitivity

- changes in skin temperature

- changes in skin colour: often blotchy, purple, pale or red

- changes in skin texture: shiny and thin, and sometimes excessively sweaty

- changes in nail and hair growth patterns

- swelling and stiffness in affected joints

- motor disability, with decreased ability to move the affected body part

- Often the pain spreads to include the entire arm or leg,

even though the initiating injury might have been only to a finger or toe. Pain can sometimes even travel to the opposite extremity. It may be heightened by emotional stress.

CRPS is an extreme example of facilitation which has spread to affect the sympathetic nervous system. Many clients, however, exhibit much less obvious signs. To really understand the process of facilitation and how it works, it is a good idea to have charts of the both the sympathetic and parasympathetic nervous systems which illustrate what might be affecting what. There are various points to be borne in mind:

- Sympathetic nerves arise from spinal cord segments T1 to L2. Therefore facilitation in any of these spinal segments is likely to result in somato-visceral or viscero-somatic loops, in other words inflamed tissue affecting organs or inflamed organs affecting tissue.

- As there is no direct neural connection between cervical nerve roots or lower lumbar nerve roots and the viscera, facilitation of these segments will not spread to the viscera.

- Parasympathetic nerves to the viscera arise from the cranium (the Vagus nerve) and from the sacrum. Therefore sacral spinal cord segments in the lower part of the spinal cord (around T12 to L1 called the conus medullaris and lumbar enlargement) may be involved in parasympathetic facilitation of pelvic organs.

- In the adult the spinal cord is considerably shorter than the vertebral column. The cord typically ends between L1 and L2 at the lumbar enlargement and Conus medullaris. This is why the kidney procedure can be helpful for most chronic back pain or any chronic condition affecting the lower part of the body.

- Vertebral subluxation may cause nerve irritation or nerve entrapment. This may lead to spinal facilitation. The level of subluxation will be considerably lower e.g. L5 than the facilitated cord segment around T11/12.

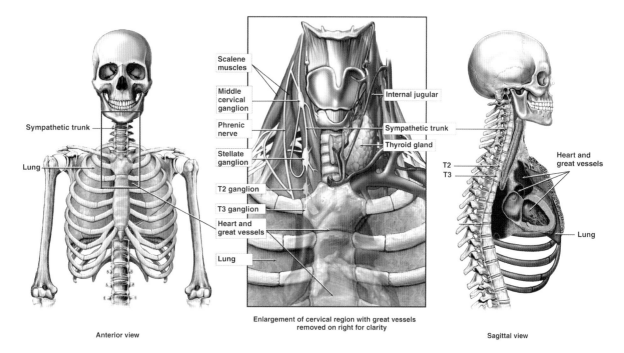

Scalene muscles

Middle cervical ganglion

Phrenic nerve

Stellate ganglion

T2 ganglion

T3 ganglion

Heart and great vessels

Lung

Internal jugular

Sympathetic trunk

Thyroid gland

Sympathetic trunk

Lung

T2
T3

Heart and great vessels

Lung

Enlargement of cervical region with great vessels removed on right for clarity

Anterior view

Sagittal view

- Pain in the distribution of a nerve and altered sensation (especially hypersensitivity) may need to be tracked to the appropriate spinal cord segment. For example: pain in the knee, L3 nerve root and T11 spinal cord segment.

- There may be divergence of sensory input into the spinal cord spanning at least three segments, e.g. if T12 segment is facilitated, the facilitation may include T11 and L1.

- Dermatomes, myotomes and scleratomes are areas of skin, muscle, and bone respectively, all derived from the same somite. A dermatome, myotome and scleratome is innervated from the same cord segment by a common nerve root. When a segment becomes facilitated, painful stimuli in any one somite component, e.g. the scleratome, may be perceived as pain in all three components. This is why a patient may experience sensitivity or numbness affecting the skin around a particular area whilst at the same time feeling a deep muscle and/or 'bony' type pain in a slightly different area.

- Scar tissue and adhesions may need to be addressed directly through work as described in Section 1. Scar tissue can hold strong 'tissue memory' and needs to be approached with sensitivity. Deep scar tissue can also be addressed by working with intention and doing appropriate Bowen moves over the skin. In this case it can be helpful to visualise the scar even if it is not apparent.

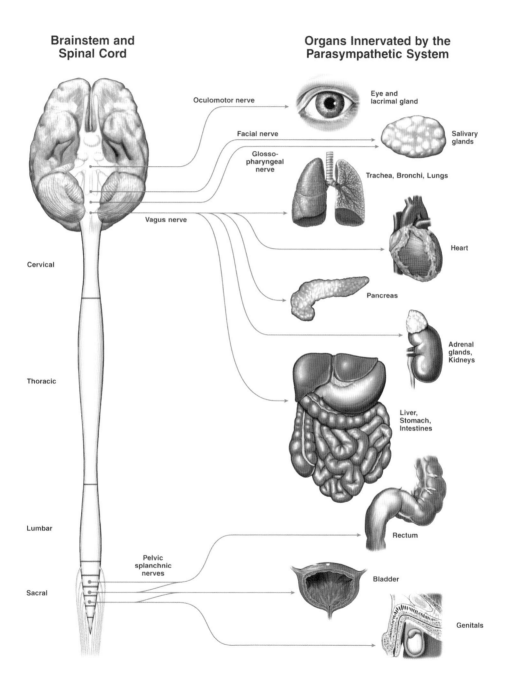

Brainstem and Spinal Cord

Organs Innervated by the Parasympathetic System

Oculomotor nerve — Eye and lacrimal gland

Facial nerve

Glosso-pharyngeal nerve — Salivary glands

Trachea, Bronchi, Lungs

Vagus nerve

Heart

Cervical

Pancreas

Adrenal glands, Kidneys

Thoracic

Liver, Stomach, Intestines

Rectum

Lumbar

Pelvic splanchnic nerves

Bladder

Sacral

Genitals

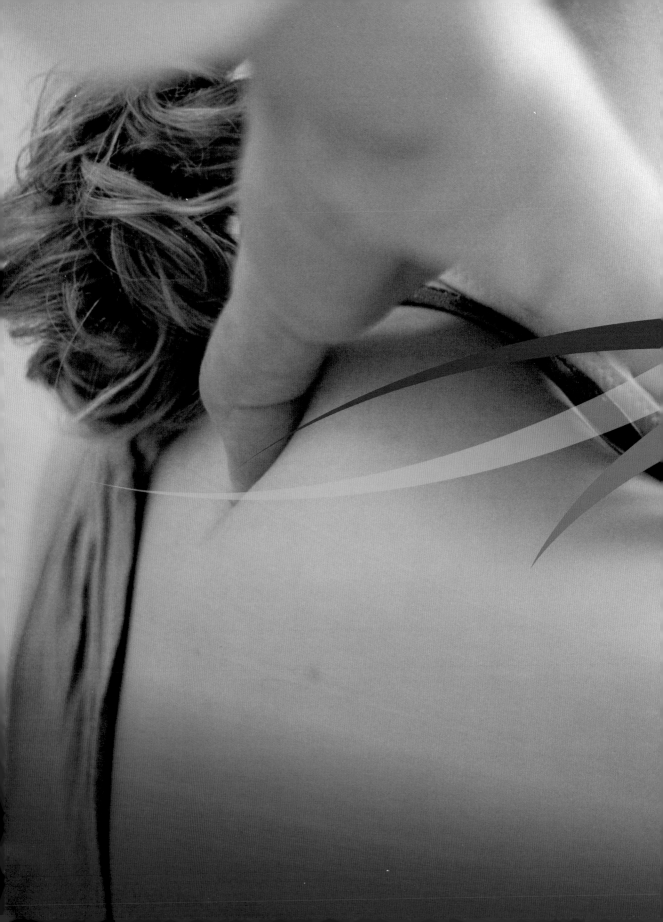

the procedures

Chapter 9

The Procedures

Although nowadays Bowen moves tend to be grouped together in 'procedures', historically this arose from observation of certain sequences of moves that Tom Bowen developed in his clinic. However, if Tom hit a situation with a client where they didn't respond, he would often 'borrow' moves from other procedures and experiment with different combinations of moves. For example, some of the moves around the neck are used in the extra moves for the shoulder that are taken from the elbow work and BRM 3.

Although certain procedures have names like the 'Frozen Shoulder' procedure or the 'Kidney' procedure, these relate much more to where the moves are performed on the body rather than a narrow prescription as to what they are for.

Take the Kidney Procedure, for example. Although a supero-lateral move is performed towards the kidneys on both sides (lateral moves tend to be more energising than medial moves), work in this area has a profound effect not just on the function of the kidney (a desire to urinate is often the result of the kidney procedure), but the sympathetic nervous system, the spinal cord and the adrenal glands.

At the level at which these moves are performed lies two important areas of the spinal cord called the conus medullaris and the lumbar enlargement. It is here (around T12 in the adult) that all the spinal nerve roots from the lower part of the body, including the legs, lower abdomen and pelvic floor region, converge and enter the spinal cord.

A lot of information is processed here, as in any spinal segment, before being conveyed to various areas of the brain such as the cerebellum and vestibular system via the spinal nerve tracts. Hypersensitivity in the conus medullaris (see chapter on nerve facilitation), which may derive from old injuries in any of the area of the lower body served by the sensory nerves, can cause muscle spasming or malfunction in any of the abdominal organs.

The kidney procedure is highly effective at reducing this facilitation in the spinal cord, leading to a reduction in sensitivity of muscle tissue (as in Fibromyalgia), a lessening of muscle spasming and improved organ function.

Reactions

Anyone who has received a Bowen treatment will recognise the distinctive waits or gaps between certain sets of moves that are the characteristic of the work.

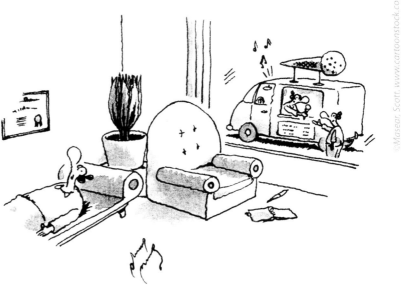

"People aren't very sensitive about my abandonment issues."

For the new practitioner, this can take some getting used to. It feels initially slightly unnatural to abandon one's client, especially on a first session just when one is just getting to know them!

However, there are good physiological and energetic reasons for doing this. The important thing for most new practitioners to realise is that these gaps in the treatment are not rigidly 2 minutes (although a minimum of 2 minutes is generally recommended), but can be variable (a bit like a train timetable – they don't always run strictly to time!).

Tom Bowen would always give plenty of time for any reaction that a client might be experiencing to settle down before moving on to complete a particular procedure or move on to a new one.

The reason for this is that the reactions the body displays as it goes through a process of release and integration happen mostly through the autonomic nervous system and it is very important that this is given time to complete its natural cycle.

Autonomic reactions have distinct tell-tale signs. These might vary from the client feeling hot or cold (sometimes in just one area of the body), tearful, tingly or sweaty etc. Sometimes the reactions can be quite subtle but are nearly always observable if one knows what to look for.

Reactions occur as the autonomic (self-regulating) nervous system processes held charge through either the sympathetic or the parasympathetic system. Occasionally, reactions happen through both systems at the same time (for example a feeling of wanting to move but feeling frozen at the same time) and this can feel quite confusing for the client.

To really understand the way the sympathetic and the parasympathetic systems work in the body, it is worth reading the book *Autonomic Nerves* by Wilson-Pauwels. To keep it simple, the reactions one might observe or the client might experience fall into two distinct categories:

Sympathetic Responses   Parasympathetic Responses

Sympathetic Responses	Parasympathetic Responses
Feeling hot	Feeling cold
Tingling	Numbness, feeling frozen
Trembling	Goose bumps
Pupils dilated	Pupils constricted and small
Flushing in the skin	Whiteness or clamminess
Heart rate speeding up	Stomach gurgling
Feeling wide awake	Feeling sleepy
Getting upset	Gentle, releasing tears
Wanting to move	Feeling withdrawn, not wanting to communicate
Heart rate rising	Feeling disassociated or 'out of it'
Breathing speeding up	Difficulty in orienting to where they are when they get up

Occasionally, especially when you 'hit the spot' with a particular procedure, responses can be very strong. It is possible for someone to experience extreme coldness, a feeling of not being able to move, feeling hot, or even panic, sometimes together with with a flooding of memories about an old injury or operation. In these situations it is vital to stay with the client and re-assure them that it is just a natural process of release and that it will soon calm down.

Reactions like this can be unfamiliar to the person and just an explanation of the way in which the autonomic nervous system processes held charge is very helpful for them. Strong reactions can occur particularly when working on scar tissue, as there are often emotional associations (for example fear) held within the area. Assessing the client's ability to cope with strong reactions is vital otherwise you risk just stirring things up and re-traumatising someone.

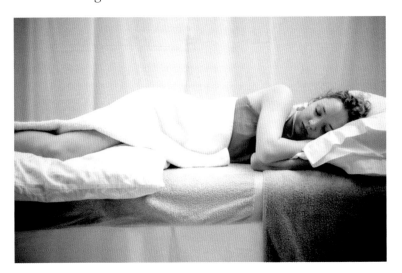

When the body re-experiences a traumatic event it has a physiological tendency to 'think' that whatever happened in the past is happening all over again. If you stir things up in this way you risk the client becoming confused, upset or even depressed because they cannot differentiate past experience from present reality. The kind of situations that might trigger this response are if you are working on scar tissue, areas around operations, in cases where someone has had a physical attack or experienced a whiplash injury.

The main things that counter-act adverse reactions are to make sure the person is resourced (possibly by doing the 'feeling good' exercise), slow things down (for example by getting them to take some good deep breaths) and try and keep them as aware as possible of physical sensation in their body (for example the sensation of contact with the couch). This allows the nervous system to process held trauma in present time, which is the only way it can do it successfully. To understand this process I recommend reading Peter Levine's book *Waking the Tiger* or if you are working with children, his book *Trauma through a Child's Eyes*. For a client to understand how their autonomic nervous system works, particularly if they are having strong emotional reactions to the treatment, can be invaluable and will make it much more likely that they will stay the course of treatment if things get tough.

Mind the Gap

In order for healing to take place, what is important is that this natural releasing process of the autonomic nervous system is not interrupted otherwise it will not be able to re-balance and come to a state of equilibrium.

For this to happen, as long as the client is not having a strong reaction, it is much better if the practitioner is out of the room. This way the patient can fully relax and there is no possibility that this process will be interrupted by any unnecessary chit-chat. Besides, most clients (particularly in England!) feel awkward about being in the same room as someone and not talking to them.

Energetically, it is also much easier on the practitioner. As things are released during the course of a treatment, it is very easy for the open practitioner to become something of a 'sponge' and even occasionally take on unsavoury sensations. I know a number of practitioners who 'take on' illnesses from their clients and end up with headaches or shoulder pains at the end of the day. This is not helpful for the client or the practitioner, and being out of the energy field of the client as their body goes through a process of release helps to avoid this.

The scientist Rupert Sheldrake has shown through experiments described in his book *The Sense of Being Stared At and Other Aspects of the Extended Mind* that when people are being observed, whether they are consciously aware of it or not, their brain-waves exhibit signs of alertness that are not conducive to relaxation. Indeed, being observed alerts areas of the brain (particularly the pre-frontal cortex) that interfere with the natural ability of the more primitive areas of the brain to settle and process information without interference.

One of the most interesting discoveries to come out of quantum physics concerns the effect of observation, intent and presence on the activity of matter. From experiments involving the observations of atoms undertaken in 1989 by Wayne Itano and his colleagues at the National Institute of Standards and Technology in Boulder, Colorado, described in Dr Fred Alan Wolf's book *The Dreaming Universe* (Simon and Schuster, 1994), it would appear that sub-atomic particles display an 'awareness' of some kind that is sensitive to observation.

Certainly, the pioneering work of Dr Masaru Emoto has shown the effect of thought on matter with startling clarity. Any practitioner who has seen his book *Hidden Messages in Water* cannot fail to realise the importance of positive thought and words when treating clients and the effect of intent on the very substance of our being.

'Absent' and 'Surrogate' Bowen
One of the more difficult aspects of Bowen for the rational mind to understand is the concept of working at a distance or 'absent' work.

In many healing traditions and in the field of Radionics in particular, the phenomenon of healing at a distance has been well documented and proven to have a beneficial effect, not only on human beings but also animals and even crops. Columbia University's study to see whether prayer affected the success of IVF treatment bears this out: (Does Prayer Influence the Success of in Vitro Fertilization–Embryo Transfer? *Report of a Masked, Randomized Trial* - Kwang Y. Cha, M.D., Daniel P. Wirth, J.D., M.S., and Rogerio A. Lobo, M.D.).

The world of quantum physics may help here as well, in that many experiments have shown the power of intent on observable phenomena such as the activity of atoms. Intent rather than intention or expectation would appear to be important here in that the appropriate action must also be involved.

Many practitioners have found that when performing absent Bowen it is much better to set up a pre-arranged time with your absent client and for the practitioner to dedicate that time actively performing the moves with focused intent, possibly on an inanimate object. Certainly in my experience, this has worked extremely well, sometimes even better than performing the moves on a person who is physically present.

Surrogate Bowen is usually performed in situations where it is impossible to work on a client directly, perhaps because they have an infectious skin condition or they have a limb in plaster etc. Here, a surrogate person is used who is healthy, and the moves are performed on that person with the intention of treating the client. Some contact between the surrogate and the client seems to be helpful when working like this. Although again, this concept may seem alien to many of a 'scientific' mind, this process has been used in mainstream practices such as chiropractic for many years with recognised benefits.

Chapter *10*

The Lower Body

The Basic Relaxation Moves 1 (page 1)

The Lower back procedure is a pre-requisite for most other lower body work and rightly so. It affects all the major fascial relationships in the body and for this reason it is always suggested to start at the lower back before moving on to upper body work.

The significance of the position of the first two moves has already been mentioned but it is also interesting that they are made at an area where several layers of fascia come together (a bit like the layers of a good lasagne). This area is called the Thoracolumbar fascia and it is at this point that many structural stress lines come together to create a strong loading area for the tissues. It is also a junction (rather like a motorway interchange) where impulses from Bowen moves can travel in many directions (mostly inferior/superior, but also supero-laterally up the latissimus fasica).

Tom Bowen, in his own enigmatic way, described how these moves send energy deep into the body, to the very bony tissue. Certainly my experience of these first two moves is that it starts a powerful process of releasing healing potency centred around the sacrum.

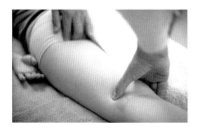 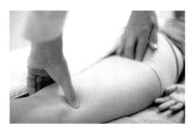 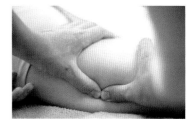

The next two moves are performed over the edge of the gluteus maximus, medius and minimus, as well as the edge of an important fascial band that comes up from the knee and connects with the whole Gluteal fascia.

The moves behind the knee are unusual in that they work directly over a nerve – the common peroneal nerve, which is a branch of the sciatic – as well as the fascia. Because there is a holding point at the heads of the Biceps Femoris and the

Semitendinosus, the impulse is in effect kept firmly within the fascia of the hamstring group.

The following moves over the Iliotibial tract go over one of the most well-defined and structurally loaded areas of the body. A common area for 'holding patterns', this move sends impulses right through the fascial system from the foot to the head.

The Psoas

The psoas is (or are, as there are two of them) one of the core muscles in the body, not only in terms of posture but also on an emotional and psychological level. The psoas is one of those muscles in the body that is inextricably linked to our primal instincts for survival and protection. It is the muscle which will curl us up into a ball if we are threatened or if there is a danger we might fall. Hence it can often hold emotions such as fear,

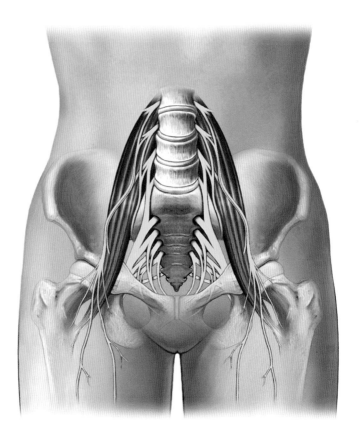

particularly when there is a perception that we might die, as can happen in car accidents or physical attack. You will often find, for example, that people who have been abused have chronically tight psoas muscles.

The Psoas group of muscles is often called the ilio-psoas because it consists of three core muscles:

1. The Psoas Major, which attaches on to the transverse processes of T12 and the lumbar vertebrae and inserts on to the lesser trochanter of the femur

2. The psoas minor, which shares a common attachment on to the vertebrae and then attaches on to the inguinal ligament

3. The iliacus, which attaches on to the iliac crest and then the lesser trochanter.

The shape of the psoas in terms of structural importance is basically triangular with its apex at T12.

Interestingly, the trapezius also forms two triangular shapes (basically a diamond), with one of its apices at T12 and the other at the base of the occiput.

Structurally, tightness through the psoas will often be reflected as a compensation pattern in the sterno-cleido-mastoid (SCM) muscle on either side, probably because both the psoas and the SCM muscles have very similar angles in the body. Whiplash injuries also tend to affect the psoas.

Most importantly, the psoas has direct muscle and fascial connections with the respiratory diaphragm. If you tune into your own psoas and cough you will feel this connection right down to the top of the inside of your femurs. This is why coughing and sneezing can have such an effect on the lumbar spine.

It is possible to palpate the common insertion of these three muscles at the lesser trochanter. Try this in the bath – bring your foot up and allow your knee to fall out to rest on the side of

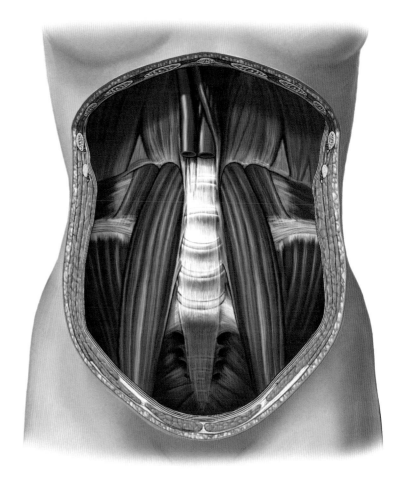

the bath so that the plantar aspect of your foot is resting on the inside of your other leg, more or less level with your knee.

Using your middle finger, feel for your adductor and gracilis muscles which attach on to your pubic bone on the middle of the inside of your leg. In this position these muscles will be quite tight and prominent.

Following the line of your inguinal ligament come out laterally about one inch and press directly down towards the floor. You should feel the insertion of the psoas at this point. It will probably feel quite tender.

Practitioners have found that with some clients it is counter-productive to attempt to get the psoas to release by working on it directly and that it is better to take the softly, softly approach by working on it indirectly.

The constructive rest position

One of the most effective things a patient can do for themselves is to adopt the constructive rest position on a daily basis for about 15 – 20 minutes a day. This is one of the best and most non-invasive ways of allowing the psoas to correct itself.

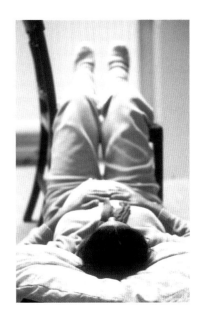

This is also one of the best exercises to do during pregnancy because a well-toned psoas muscle is essential for a comfortable pregnancy and childbirth. Women who are holding a lot of anxiety about the pregnancy or impending birth will tend to contract into their psoas muscles. This in turn tends to push the baby more anterior, thereby creating less space for it in the womb as well as constricting the pelvic outlet during birth. Very often a mum who has a very prominent 'bump' during the later stages of the pregnancy will have tight psoas muscles.

If you are going to suggest this position during pregnancy the mum does have to be supported through the back so that the baby doesn't press on the Vena Cava or the Aorta, and some midwives will also suggest that they are supported lightly through one side of the body so they are slightly tilted. Get your mother-to-be to ask her midwife for advice on this.

Although essentially very simple, this position can also bring up a lot of strong feelings for some people, perhaps feelings of fear or even sensations of trembling or shaking. It is a good idea, therefore, to go through some simple centering and resourcing exercises with your client before suggesting this exercise. (See chapter on resourcing).

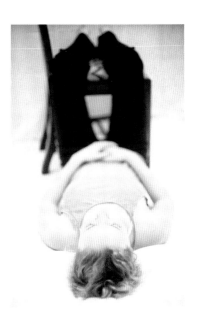

There are a number of implications for having a tight psoas on one side or the other. Firstly, the psoas muscles naturally have a massaging effect on the internal organs as we move around the kidneys, womb, liver, stomach etc. If it is tight there is more likelihood for adhesions and lack of mobility generally for the abdominal organs.

The effect on breathing has already been noted because of its direct link with the diaphragm, but tightness through these muscles will also effect the structures that pass through the diaphragm – the oesophagus, the vagus nerve, the vena cava and the aorta, restricting their ability to function freely.

Because the psoas attaches on to the transverse processes of the lumbar vertebrae, there is a lot of scope for rotational patterns to be fed into the vertebrae and create torsion through the vertebral bodies and intervertebral discs. Hence the psoas is so often implicated in disc problems.

Some practitioners who work with newborns have found that some are born with chronically tight psoas muscles. Whether this might be as a result of the baby trying instinctively to lessen the effect of living in a toxic womb environment as some practitioners have claimed, I don't know, but it certainly will tend to produce a very colicky baby.

Car Accidents

Car accidents can have a particularly devastating effect on the psoas. Seat belts have had an amazing success in saving huge numbers of lives but from the point of view of the poor old psoas they can be a bad thing.

What tends to happen is that during an impact the psoas will instinctively contract to protect the abdominal organs. Because the person is usually wearing a seat belt this contractive reaction is halted and can often result in a frozen contraction of the psoas, mostly on the side of the shoulder strap (on the left for the passenger, on the right for the driver in the UK). This situation is the reverse in the rest of Europe where they drive on the opposite side of the road.

To compound matters, the psoas in this situation will often also hold 'tissue memory' relating to the impact and make it all the more difficult for someone to let go of, particularly if the accident was traumatic. This is why a very careful, non-invasive approach is essential.

However, through use of the constructive rest position, the protocol outlined below and an explanation to the client, all this can be remedied fairly swiftly in most cases. Liz Koch's excellent books on the psoas can be a very useful resource for clients and practitioners alike. Her workshops provide an invaluable insight into the importance of these muscles. (www.coreawareness.com).

Testing for psoas involvement

When someone has a tight psoas on one side or the other (or both), certain things will be apparent. Apart from a posture that involves the trunk being pulled anterior to the legs (you can see this from the position that the arms rest in when someone is starting upright – the middle finger may lie anterior to the seam of the trousers), you will notice that there is often a gap between the couch and the back of the knee as they lie down on their back. They will often need a support under their knee to feel comfortable.

There will usually be an exaggerated lordosis of the lumbar spine (the natural curvature in the lumbar area will be more pronounced) or there may be a marked rotation of any or all of the lumbar vertebrae.

Working with the psoas

Although there is a very good advanced move for the Psoas, direct manipulation is not always advisable as it can make the psoas go into protective mode or into spasm if the person is holding on to a strong protective pattern. The following protocol has been found to be highly effective at addressing psoas issues:

BRM 1, moves 1 – 4
BRM 2, moves 1 – 4 (top stoppers) and moves 9 – 16
Kidney
Lower Respiratory moves 3 – 5
Pelvis

The work up the mid-back (moves 9 – 16 and kidney) addresses the attachments of the psoas onto the lumbar vertebrae and T12. The respiratory moves on the front of the body address the diaphragm and act as 'stoppers' to contain the work whilst the pelvic procedure addresses the psoas by working the top of the femur close to the lesser trochanter. Encourage your client to use the constructive rest position every day for around 20 minutes

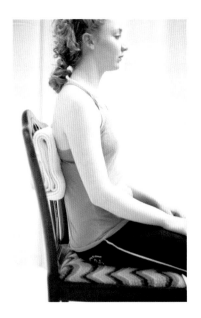

if possible. See if they are able to tune into their psoas (you can show them where it is on a diagram) and get them to imagine it softening and lengthening. Simply bringing an awareness to these muscles can have a greatly beneficial effect.

Ergonomic considerations

The psoas will become tight and congested through driving and sitting at a desk. This can be eased by sitting with one's hip joints around 5 cm higher than one's knees. The use of a wedge cushion can help with this. It is also important to have one's feet (the plantar aspect) flat on the ground.

The Coccyx

The coccyx procedure is one of the most powerful in the Bowen repertoire even though it only involves two light moves. The first is over the centre of the coccyx and the other (which Mr Bowen used to say 'locked in' the first move) is over the rectus abdominus fascia.

There are several reasons why this move is powerful. For a start, the coccyx is a crucial area for balancing the autonomic nervous system. Both the sympathetic and the parasympathetic nervous systems have important ganglia and nerve pathways that go close to the coccyx.

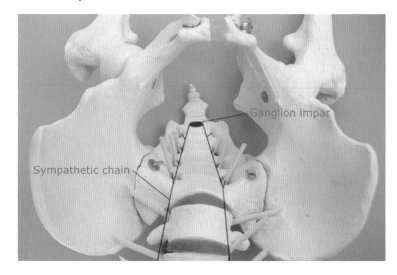

The sympathetic nervous system consists of a chain of very fine nerves which run down either side of the spine from controlling nuclei in the brain stem. These two chains have an important junction at the top of the coccyx called the ganglion of impar (or the imperial ganglion).

The parasympathetic system also has nerve pathways which originate close to the coccyx and control the bladder, lower bowel and reproductive systems. All these parts rely on a perfect balance to work properly and there is no doubt that the coccyx procedure helps in this. For example, control of the bladder is mediated by the sympathetic nerves which allow the bladder to hold on when there is no toilet in sight on the M25, whilst the parasympathetic nerve supply allows urination.

Sexual activity depends on the same balance – parasympathetic activation is necessary for arousal whilst orgasm is a sympathetic response. It is not surprising then that anxiety (which comes from an overactive sympathetic nervous system) will decrease libido and may result in erectile problems in men, or frigidity.

The coccyx is the only place in the body where the three layers of membrane that surround the brain and spinal cord (the dura, arachnoid and pia) come together (see chapter on the dura). The first move of the coccyx procedure moves right over this and sends an impulse all the way up the spinal cord to the anterior attachment of the dura at the ethmoid (the third eye, just between and above the eyes, also known as the ajna chakra).

There are interesting variations on the coccyx procedure – for example when it is used for bedwetting children, two extra holding points are used either side of the spine to contain the work. Interestingly, these two holding points correspond to a primitive reflex in babies called the Spinal Galant reflex which is supposed to be inhibited at around 4 months but may still be present up to around 10 months. One of the ways one can observe if this reflex is still active is to stroke down the erector spinae either side of the spine – this will elicit urination if the reflex is still active. This procedure could well help in the inhibition of this reflex in bedwetting children, where the reflex is still active.

The coccyx procedure has also been found to be effective in working with people with disc problems. One of the reasons for this might be that as mentioned in the chapter on embryology the practitioner is moving over the filament terminalis which is attached to the highly fluid membranes surrounding the spinal cord. It could be that this move awakens a tissue memory of the notochord, whose remnants can be found in the centre of the inter-vertebral discs, and thereby encourages a re-orientation of the body towards the midline. One interesting feature of the inter-vertebral discs is that they have collagen fibres running vertically through them. This means that impulses will tend to travel strongly through them in a inferior – superior direction.

Other variations of the coccyx procedure include working both sides of the coccyx (with a 20 minute break in between) to address piriformis pain.

The Pelvis

The pelvic work is one of the most frequently performed 'procedures' in the Bowen repertoire. It promotes massive change through the whole pelvic bowl and influences the positioning of the pelvis in relation to the rest of the body.

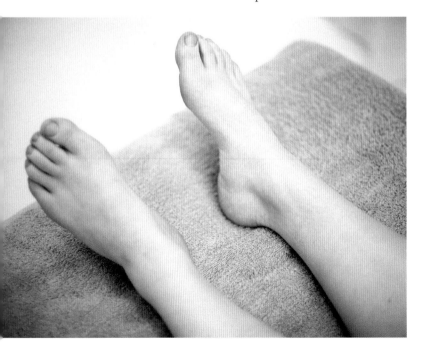

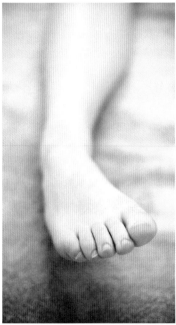

The necessity for performing the pelvic procedure can be ascertained by observing the client lying on their back: are their ankles at the same level; is there an angle between the foot and the tibia/fibula?

There are many possibilities for the pelvis to become 'out of place'. Rotational patterns may be due to psoas involvement, whereas a 'tipping backwards' of the pelvis, resulting in a lessening of the natural lordosis of the lumbar spine, maybe because of tightness through the hamstrings. In most cases there are combinations of different factors affecting the position of the pelvis and its related impact on everything above and below it. Where the pelvic procedure really comes into its own is in cases of apparent leg-length discrepancy and issues with the pelvic bowl in general.

The pelvic procedure is interesting in that it works mostly on the front fascial relationship (or superficial front line that Tom Myers identifies) and muscles controlled by the femoral nerve. Because the last move goes over the attachment of the psoas minor as well as close to the femoral nerve, artery and vein, this procedure has a massive effect on blood and nerve supply to the leg as well as on the lymphatic system.

The Hamstrings

Tightness through the hamstrings will tend to pull down on the ischial tuberosity (sitting bone) and create stiffness through the lower back. Specifically it can create a lack of natural lordosis in the lumbar area and restrictions in the sacro-iliac joints.

Interestingly, in many four legged animals, including horses, part of the hamstring group attaches straight on to the sacrum. In essence one can see the strong continuity of the fascial relationship of the hamstrings through the sacro-tuberous ligament and the fascia around the erector spinae muscles.

Energetically, the intention of the hamstring procedure is to separate these two groups of muscles so that they can work independently of each other. Many times, especially if someone

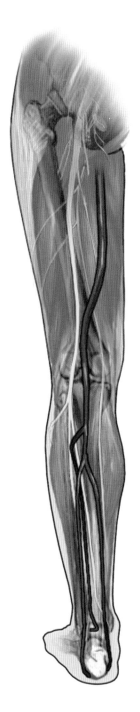

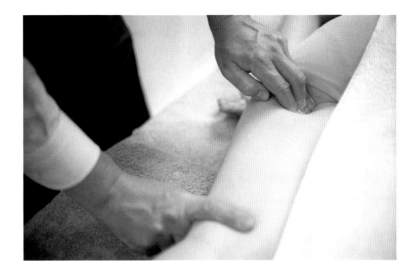

does a lot of exercise like jogging, the biceps femoris and the semi-tendonosis can almost act as one muscle because of the adhesions between them – especially around the top of the leg towards the gluteal fold. This creates a lack of mobility right the way through the fascial tract.

The straight leg raise test is useful for ascertaining where the restrictions are coming from, and will let you know exactly where to work. Sometimes, if the restrictions are held only in the upper portion of the hamstrings, it is more appropriate to perform the 5A and 7A moves medially – this is done by having your holding point at the popliteal fossa and performing a fairly strong move medially over the heads of the hamstrings. Tom Bowen would do this if he felt there was still a holding pattern here after performing the BRM 1 procedure and allowing the body to settle for five minutes. He called the indication that this area needed addressing a 'stigma'.

Where restrictions are felt further down the leg it might be appropriate to concentrate more on the gastrocnemius muscles by doing the knee procedure. This will become clear when you do the straight leg raise test.

The Sacrum

The test for sacro-iliac restriction has been discussed in the chapter on assessment. What is really interesting is to look also at how these restrictions can affect the neck. Anyone with a sacro-iliac restriction will have a related neck restriction on the opposite side. This is partly because of the fascial connections between the sacrum and the neck, but also because of the strong attachments of the dural membrane at centre of the sacrum (S2) and the top of the neck.

It can be fun to do the sacrum test and then ask the client to turn their head slowly left and right. Notice if their neck improves after doing the sacral procedure – they will be amazed! Ninety-five percent of the time there will be some improvement in the neck. This is not to say that there may not be some other issue affecting the neck locally, but the sacral procedure should help.

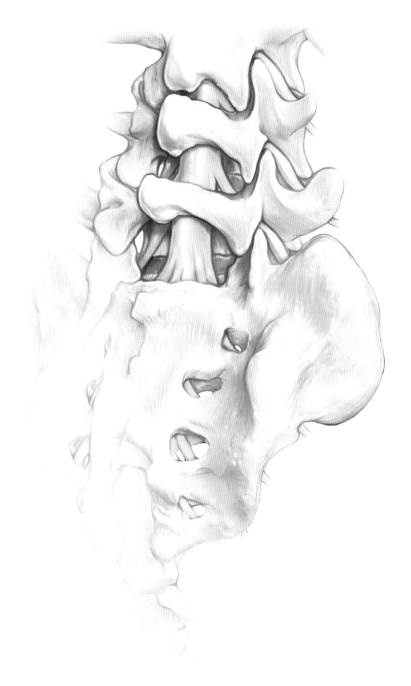

The other possibility is that there may be some hyper-mobility in the sacro-iliac joints – this might be after someone has done a lot of yoga or has had repeated chiropractic or osteopathic manipulation. The essential thing in this situation is to try and get some stability back into the area. Specific Pilates exercises to strengthen the ligaments and core muscles, together with Chi Kung and homeopathic remedies might be needed before the area becomes stable enough to be able to hold Bowen work long–term.

The sacral moves themselves are the epitome of minimalism. Although Tom Bowen often used to work on one side only (especially when working on women in the later stages of pregnancy), we usually now teach working both sides as so often people hold some form of restriction there as well.

The first move goes over the sacro-tuberous ligament (a ligament capable of holding over 7000 kilos of strain – and we have two of them!). What is interesting is the position that Tom Bowen recommended because it allows much better access to the ligament itself than if they were lying on their front. Getting the client to take their weight through their arms also shifts the weight from the sacro-iliac joints - if you think that most four-legged animals take two thirds of their body weight through their front legs, that's how you want them to be. I don't recommend you tell your clients to stand like a dog, but that is what you want!

The second move of the sacrum involves having a holding point at the top of the sacro-tuberous ligament that effectively inhibits the impulse of the move travelling down the leg and concentrates the work energetically in the ligaments that suspend the sacrum between the wings of the ilia. What is important here is to feel a definite pulse in the holding point as you do the second move.

The construction of the whole pelvis is fascinating from a structural engineering point of view, with its tension patterns held through the inguinal ligaments and the extreme forces held in the ligaments holding the sacrum in place. Here, almost more than anywhere else in the body, one can see how the human body has had to adapt to an upright posture and why it is prone to problems in the lower back and sacrum. The genius of the moves that Tom Bowen developed are clear to see, when one observes the almost instantaneous changes that occur after the sacral procedure.

The Kidneys

The symptoms of a kidney infection may include feeling distinctly unwell, pain when urinating or even blood in the urine.

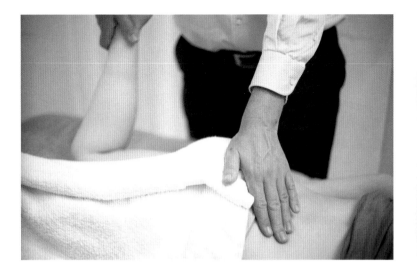

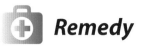

Kidney Cleanse

Tom Bowen would advise his patients to take 2 slices of raw beetroot per day for a maximum of 14 days. This can be in the form of grating it in salad or juicing it. It is worth advising your client that they may observe some red staining of stools and urine. Advice should always be taken from their doctor or pharmacist on possible contra-indications if taking medication (for example antibiotics)

Any situation like this needs to be treated urgently and you need to tell your client to see a doctor immediately. Untreated kidney infections can lead to serious complications and kidney damage.

However, the kidney procedure is indicated for many more situations than just conditions affecting the kidneys themselves. It can be used to address dizziness, adrenal problems, oedema, lymphatic issues and, as mentioned before, chronic pain and hyper-sensitivity.

The position that Tom Bowen suggested for the client is interesting in that it isolates the various layers of fascia around the upper lumbar. By flexing the leg and taking it out laterally

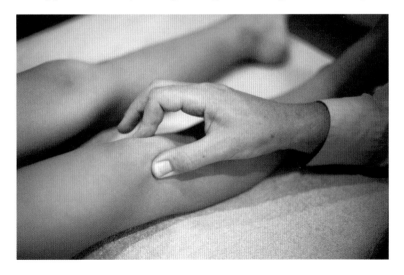

it stresses the latissimus fascia, thereby allowing the impulses created by the move to travel clearly in one direction.

The Knee

The knee procedure is quite complex and involves work on many different components of the leg – ligaments, muscles and nerves. The straight leg raise test will show you if there is any myofascial restriction that can be isolated – sometimes these can be felt in the Achilles tendon or even in the plantar aspect of the foot.

However, the knee procedure is excellent for many other types of condition including oedema, cruciate ligament damage, arthritis and non-resolving back pain. The knee will tend to 'get it in the neck' if there is any foot, ankle or pelvic imbalance as it will have to deal with the strong compensation patterns that result. It is always worth checking these aspects as well and treat accordingly.

The various moves of the knee procedure effect the retinacular ligaments, the vastus medialis, the gastrocnemius, the achilles tendon and the tibial nerve. Tom Bowen would also frequently apply strapping below the patella to stabilise it but this is not generally taught these days. The soda pack that he developed is so effective at draining fluid off joints, and the knee in particular, that it is now used in hospitals throughout Austria.

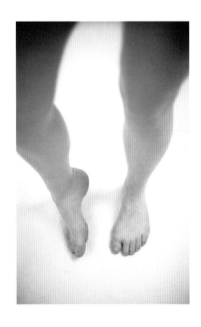

One of the most difficult moves to get right is the last move over the tibial nerve as it is easy to confuse it with other nerves on the medial aspect of the ankle. This nerve is a branch of the sciatic nerve and the move can be used in isolation to treat pain in the perineum (the spot between the genitals and the anus).

The Ankle

An interesting feature of the ankle procedure (and the associated work for hammer toes and bunions), is that it works almost exclusively by affecting the ligaments and the fascia, particularly the plantar fascia of the foot which is essentially the inferior end of the whole fascial 'train' that ends at the back of the head.

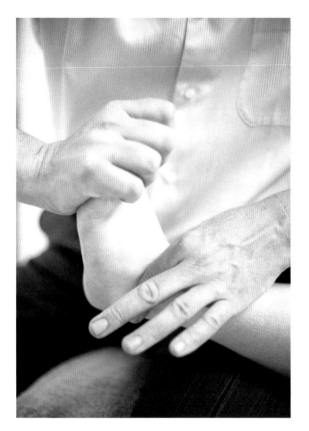

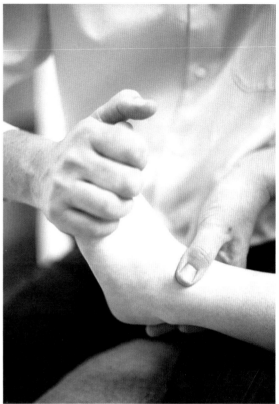

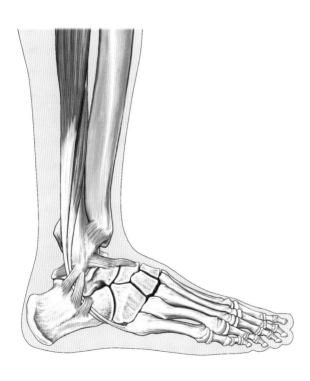

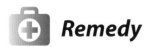

Remedy

Bunion treatment

Tom Bowen would ask his clients with bunions to soak their feet every night in warm water to which 2-3 tablespoons of Epsom Salts have been added, for at least 6 weeks. He would also suggest that after each soaking they applied a small amount of iodex ointment to the affected area. This can also be beneficial for heel spurs.

Iodex is hard to come by nowadays but some chemists may be able to make up the ointment for you. It is made up of 25% iodine (to reduce the inflammation) and 75% methyl salicylate (to break down the calcification). Be careful if your client has a thyroid problem as the iodine can interfere with their medication.

Commonly injuries occur when people go over on the outside of their foot and damage the lateral ligaments, particularly the anterior tibio-fibular ligament (ATFL).

A tendency to injure this area repeatedly is usually down to a related hip or pelvic imbalance causing undue pressure or instability on this area, and this would need to be addressed.

After addressing the retinacular ligament in the first move, the second move goes right over the ATFL in two directions. Often

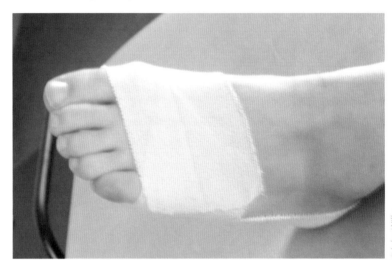

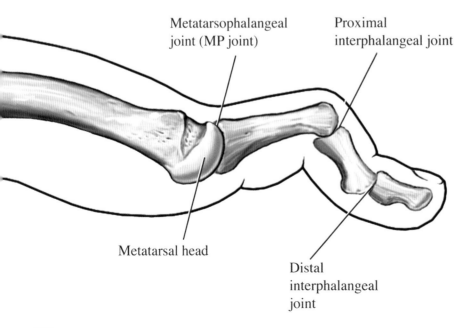

Metatarsophalangeal joint (MP joint)

Proximal interphalangeal joint

Metatarsal head

Distal interphalangeal joint

this area can be quite 'puffy' and inflamed in someone who has a tendency to injury here.

The strapping that Tom Bowen developed for Hammer Toes and Plantar Fasciitis is not taught any more in many schools of Bowen. However, both can be invaluable in allowing the foot the opportunity to repair without repeated strain being put on the area.

With the strapping for Hammer Toes, tape is applied to the underside of the foot to create a stretch through the tendons in the dorsal aspect of the foot and to straighten the toes when walking. This is highly successful in most cases of hammer toes.

The strapping for plantar fasciitis is equally effective at removing the continual stretching and contracting of the plantar fascia when walking and supporting the arch of the foot. Useful for people with 'fallen arches' this strapping also allows the foot space and time for repair after the specific moves have been applied.

Chapter 11

The Upper Body

Basic Relaxation Moves 2 (page 2)

A fundamental pre-requisite for most upper body procedures, the upper back and shoulder work includes some of the most relaxing moves in Bowen. The 'top stoppers' particularly, if done with good deep breaths (as Tom Bowen recommended), are helpful on their own if someone is distressed or in shock.

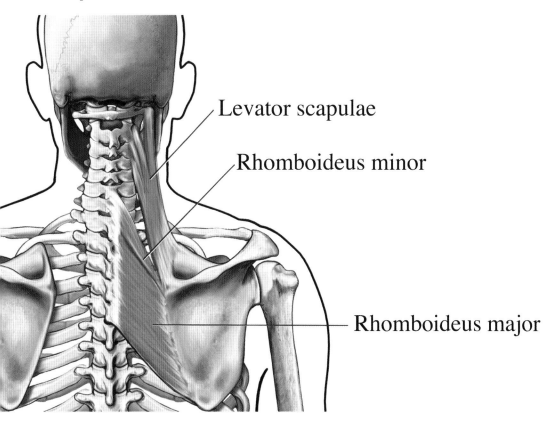

Levator scapulae

Rhomboideus minor

Rhomboideus major

The so called 'boomerang' moves around the trapezius and rhomboids can be divided into two pairs of moves and should ideally involve a nice challenge on the levator scapula muscle as well. The levator scapulae attach on to the upper part of the cervical vertebrae so the moves have a profound effect on the neck as well as a wonderful relaxing effect on the shoulders.

Tom Bowen described the moves over the latissimus dorsi muscles as the 'crowbar' moves and they can sometimes feel that tight! These moves are profoundly useful for shoulder restrictions and for any general tightness through the lower thoracic and lumbar

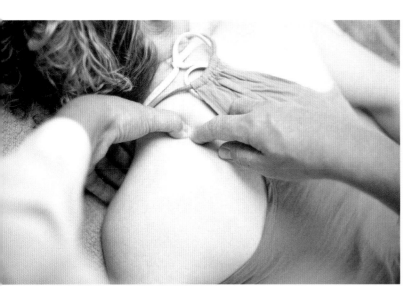

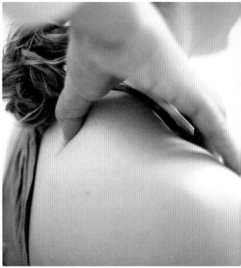

areas because of the way the muscle wraps around the back. We have talked about the effect of the alternating moves 9 – 16 up the back on the sympathetic nervous system, but I always ascertain the need for these moves by gentle palpation of the erector spinae muscles before I start a treatment, or by scanning the spine.

Basic Relaxation Moves 3 (page 3)

These moves for addressing the neck need to be performed in conjunction with the upper back and shoulder work to be really effective. The first moves go over the posterior and middle scalenes respectively. These muscles are unusual as they attach on to the cervical vertebrae and the second and first rib respectively. It is easy to miss the posterior scalene unless you take enough skin slack posteriorly first, and it should feel quite distinct if you get it right.

The moves on the occiput address the superior aspect of Tom Myers' superficial back line. If ever there was a Bowen move which needs to be done in the right place, this is it. At the back of the occiput there are several muscles overlapping each other and attaching on to the nuchal crests. The most superficial is the trapezius, which can feel quite stringy at this point. This attaches on to the most superior nuchal crests, which lie just above and

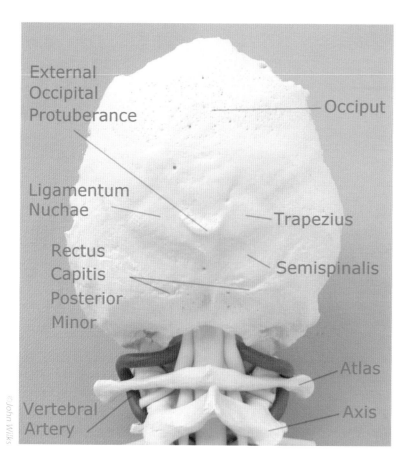

External Occipital Protuberance

Occiput

Ligamentum Nuchae

Trapezius

Rectus Capitis Posterior Minor

Semispinalis

Atlas

Vertebral Artery

Axis

©John Wilks

either side of the inion (the occipital protruberance or 'bump of knowledge').

It is here that you have two very important lymph nodes – the occipital lymph nodes. This is partly why it can be so sensitive to touch if someone's system is overloaded or toxic. Lymph nodes are innervated by sympathetic nerves, so the moves here have a direct effect on the autonomic system as well.

Just below the trapezius lies the semispinalis, which feels wider and softer to the touch. Beneath that, and a little more inferior, is the rectus capitis posterior minor which is a fascinating little muscle that attaches on to C1 (the atlas). This muscle in particular is prone to injury in situations like whiplash simply because it is so short. It was only recently discovered that the rectus capitis has the important function of pulling the dural membrane out of the way in certain neck movements. If these muscles get damaged they can atrophy, with the result that the

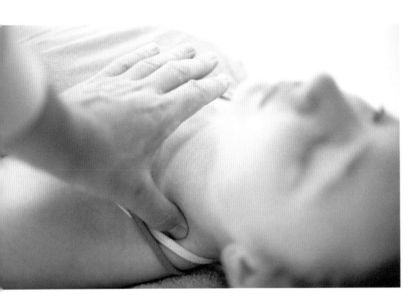
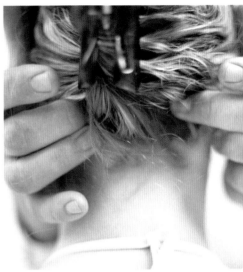

dura can become trapped and inflamed.

One way one can test the position of the rectus capitis muscle on oneself is to feel the location just lateral and inferior to the inion and, without moving your head, move your eyes left and right or up and down. You should feel a subtle movement underneath your fingers. The reason for this is because of the direct neural connection between neck movement and eye movement – part of our 'social nervous system' that Stephen Porges talks about.

The last two moves really do have a profound effect on the back fascial band and send impulses all the way down to the feet. Indeed, it is not unusual for clients to say that they felt those moves in their toes!

The variation on the neck moves that we use in the thoracic procedure (or chest pain procedure) is a study in minimalism. By performing stoppers front and back (the respiratory moves effectively act as stoppers in the front) we set up the body for sending powerful impulses right into the chest cavity.

Lower Respiratory

Many practitioners ask why the first two lateral moves on the back are performed on the right side first. The answer is somewhat mundane in that in Tom Bowen's clinic his beds were placed so that their left hand sides would be nearest to him as he entered the door. This meant it was easier to perform the right move first. When the client turned over it was then easier to perform the moves on the left side of the diaphragm first. Having said that, his explanation was that it was irrelevant which side of the back was done first but very important that the front moves over the attachments of the diaphragm were done left side first. The answers to many of these oddities we will probably never know, but it certainly keeps the various Bowen chat rooms busy!

Those first two moves of the respiratory are highly energetic and effectively direct two very strong impulses into the thoracic cavity. In some schools of Bowen a lot of emphasis is put upon the accurate positioning of these moves at a line just above the inferior angle of the scapula. Could it be that Tom considered it to be important that the moves are performed just superior to where the myofascia of the latissimus dorsi attaches on to the thoracic vertebrae? It would certainly have a very different effect in terms of where the impulses would travel if the moves were done any lower.

The importance of the moves over the attachments of the diaphragm have been noted in the section on the psoas muscles, but these moves also go over the stomach, flexures of the large intestine and the liver. The last move (which needs to be done on the full exhalation) is fascinating because it affects so many structures at the same time. It goes over some strong attachments of the diaphragm onto the xyphoid, the linea alba (a tough band of ligament and fascia which goes all the way down to the pubis), and the falciform ligament (a remnant of the umbilical vein), which goes through the liver. This could be why this move can have such a strong emotional effect as it touches on very deep tissue memories to do with connection, our first breath and coming into the world. This move on its own can also be a life-saver for anyone suffering an asthmatic attack (having first called for an ambulance of course).

The Chest (or Breast Procedure)

This simple procedure is so effective at counteracting all kinds of problems with the breast that a well-known cancer charity asked recently if it could be taught as a preventative measure to women in their classes. Essentially these moves assist lymphatic drainage from the many lymph nodes in the breast and axilla (the armpit).

The issue of how much (if at all) women should wear bras has been a hot topic ever since the 1960's. In some cultures, (particularly in countries like Greece and Turkey), girls wear bras 24 hours a day, however research (outlined in the book *Dressed to Kill: The Link between Breast Cancer and Bras* by Sydney Singer and Soma Grismaijer) shows that wearing a bra more than eight hours a day considerably increases one's chances of developing some problem in that area.

The main issues with bras, particularly if they are too tight, are that they:

- Restrict the natural movement of the breast (lymphatic flow is dependent on movement)

- Restrict the movement of lymph up through the armpit, particularly if the strap around the lateral sides of the body is tight

- Put pressure on the lymphatic duct right at the centre of the base of the breast – this is particularly true with under-wire bras

- Put pressure on trigger points in the trapezius muscles where the strap goes over the shoulder, particularly if the woman is fairly large-breasted

- Put pressure on an individual thoracic vertebra if the strap is too tight or skimpy, leading to vertebral subluxation and nerve irritation

Lymph nodes are interesting in that they each have a sympathetic nerve going to them. If someone's sympathetic system is too active then their lymphatic system will tend to be affected too.

The moves themselves are probably most effective being taught as a self-help technique. A woman can do these moves in the comfort of her own home, in the bath or lying in bed. If treating the left side (one always treats the better or least affected side first) one can use the side of the index finger of the right hand to bring the breast tissue down and do a medial move with the out breath. For the lower move, it is important to be below the centre of the breast and one can use the pad of the index finger to perform a lateral move, lifting up the breast a little to get underneath it. This move should feel slightly tender. It is much better if both these moves can be done on the exhalation.

As a preventative measure this can be done every month but if there is congestion or tenderness, then once a week is recommended. It goes without saying that a woman should be examining her breasts every month in any case and that anything unusual should be referred to a doctor immediately.

Shoulder

Tom Bowen called the shoulder work the 'Frozen Shoulder' procedure because (or so the story goes) he once had to treat a butcher who developed pain in his shoulder after carrying heavy frozen shoulders of meat on his shoulder! Hence it is much more than just a procedure for addressing classic 'frozen shoulder'.

This procedure works primarily on the deltoid muscle and fascia – first posterior and then anterior. Along with its associated procedures, BRM 2 & 3, the strangely named north, south, east, west moves and the elbow procedure, all of the fascial meridians that Tom Myers isolates as the front and back arm lines are addressed.

As mentioned in the chapter on assessment, it is vital to ascertain where exactly the nerve entrapment or fascial restriction is in order to treat effectively. Have we ruled out the possibility of referred pain from the neck, the brachial plexus, the elbow or the wrist?

The extra moves that Tom Bowen developed for non-responding

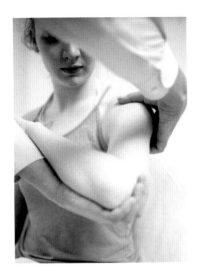

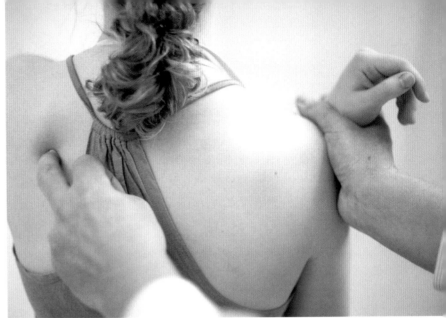

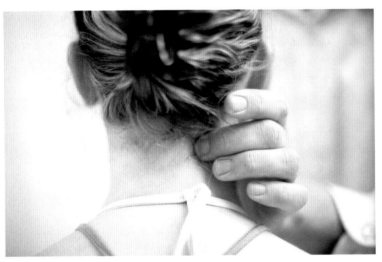

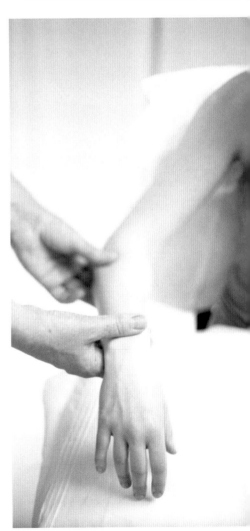

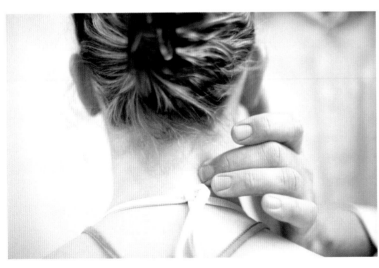

shoulder restrictions are spectacular in their effectiveness, but many are difficult to really understand, even from a study of the fascial relationships in the arm. Why is it, for example, that the last move of the neck procedure performed a little lower over the trapezius muscle, should, if used in the right situation, have such a dramatic effect on shoulder mobility?

The Upper Respiratory Temporo-Mandibular Joints (or TMJ)

Tom Bowen developed the upper respiratory procedure initially for people suffering from hayfever and other allergy-related conditions affecting the upper respiratory tract. With the addition of the TMJ work it becomes one of the most powerful procedures in the Bowen repertoire. As mentioned in the previous section, Tom Bowen was intensely interested in facial dynamics and observing facial asymmetry can be very helpful in determining if the TMJ work is indicated.

The temporo-mandibular joints themselves are one of the core bi-lateral joints in the body and structurally will tend to reflect the hip joints. They also have a profound effect on the neck, partly because when one opens one's mouth, the condyles of the mandible move anteriorly rather than just open and shut like a normal hinge joint. This means that the true centre of rotation of the jaw is actually at the second cervical vertebra, specifically the dens of C2, which is a peg-like structure around which the atlas swivels. Hence, a jaw which is out of line will directly affect the neck.

One of the remarkable effects of the Upper Respiratory and TMJ work seems to be to encourage drainage all through the neck and base of the cranium and specifically to create more space laterally. Because some very important structures pass through the jugular foramen, close behind the ear, one often observes a cascade of changes after doing this work. The jugular foramen is formed by the junction of two bones, the occiput and the temporal bone, and is therefore very susceptible to medial compressive forces, which will then restrict the outflow of blood from the cranium. Given that 95% of all the de-oxygenated blood from the cranium

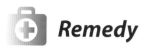

Remedy

Treating Joints

One can apply the same principles of the bunion procedure to treating fingers:

Apply gentle traction to the finger whilst at the same time making some gentle moves over the joint towards the thumb side of the hand (laterally in the anatomical position). I have used this in many cases of arthritis or 'mouse finger' to great effect. It is often helpful to address the joint above and below the affected joint as well.

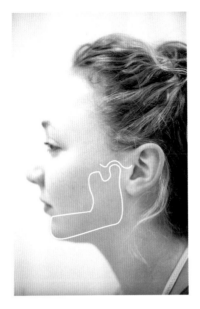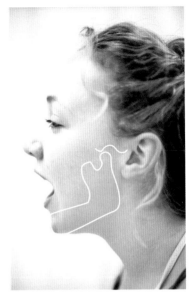
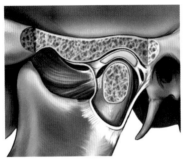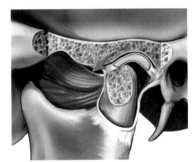

Lateral view of TMJ showing movement of the mandible

flows out through this foramen, this can be pretty major and can create symptoms like pressure headaches and general 'muzziness'.

Medial compression around the ears and temporal bones can be created by all kinds of factors – wearing glasses, holding tension through the jaw or even unresolved birth issues such as forceps delivery.

There are three pairs of cranial nerves that exit the cranium through the same passageway and are equally susceptible to compression. These are cranial nerves IX, X and XI or the Glossopharyngeal, Vagus, and Spinal Accessory nerves. They all have considerable interaction, shared anatomy and functional overlap and they share important nuclei in the brain stem which also are involved in regulating the autonomic nervous system, specifically the Dorsal Vagal Nucleus, the Solitary Tract Nucleus

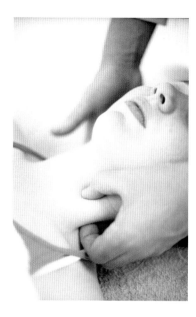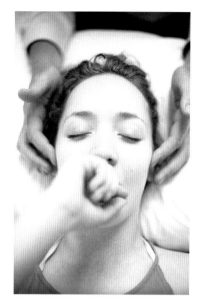

and the Nucleus Ambiguus.

One of the most interesting researchers in the field of how cranial nerves interact is Stephen Porges, professor of psychiatry at the University of Illinois in Chicago. He has developed a convincing theory he calls the Polyvagal theory, which describes the complex interaction of the cranial nerves and the autonomic nervous system together as a 'social nervous system'. He developed this theory to relate the evolutionary shift in the neural regulation of the autonomic nervous system to the range and regulation of emotion expressed and experienced by humans. His pioneering work (along with Stanley Rosenburg in Copenhagen) on autism could well provide a breakthrough in understanding and treating this complex and distressing condition.

Medial compressive forces are common and may result in a cascade of seemingly unrelated symptoms because of the action on the cranial nerves and the jugular vein. Symptoms might include:

*   Tightness or stiffness in the trapezius or sterno-cleido-mastoid muscle (in extreme cases it might result in torticollis or wry-neck) because of the effect on the accessory nerve

*   Digestive, breathing, heart or lung problems because of the

effect on the vagus nerve

- Pressure headaches, 'muzziness' in the head, or an inability to remember things

One of the reasons we tend to use the TMJ work for unresolved neck problems is because of its strong effect on the spinal accessory nerve.

This nerve is crucial in addressing head forward posture as it essentially controls the relationship between the back fascia via the trapezius and the front fascia via the sterno-cleido-mastoid.

The other major nerve to be affected by compression is the vagus nerve, which derives its name from the same latin root as vagrant, wandering throughout the body and controlling functions such as heart rate, breathing, liver, kidney, small intestine, stomach and part of the large intestine. This is the nerve which comes into play when we begin to relax. Because it is the major parasympathetic nerve in the body it will make our stomach gurgle (always a good sign) when we have a treatment.

We have already noted how imbalances in the bite will effect posture and how it is still possible to treat effectively many years after the event. However, because the forces that are often held here tend to go back a long time, several treatments may be

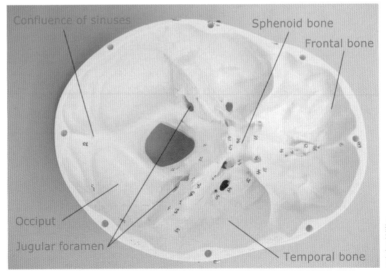

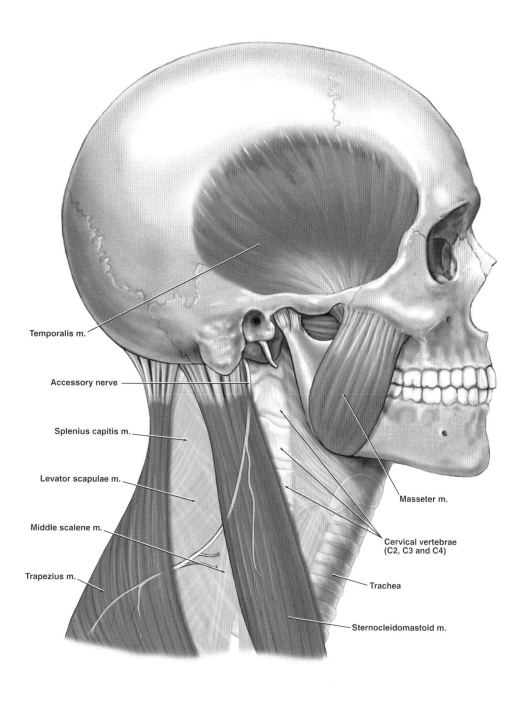

Temporalis m.

Accessory nerve

Splenius capitis m.

Levator scapulae m.

Middle scalene m.

Trapezius m.

Masseter m.

Cervical vertebrae
(C2, C3 and C4)

Trachea

Sternocleidomastoid m.

*Cranial nerve XI – the
spinal accessory*

necessary to effect a change. The advanced work which involves performing the TMJ work twice with slight variations and moving over the masseter muscle can also be highly effective in stubborn cases.

The Cranium

Previously referred to as the 'headache' procedure, these gentle moves work over the major deep relaxation points in kinesiology. Apart from invoking relaxation, these moves also effect the sinuses, can help resolve birth trauma by influencing the flow of cerebro-spinal fluid and effect the natural subtle, tide-like movements of the cranial bones.

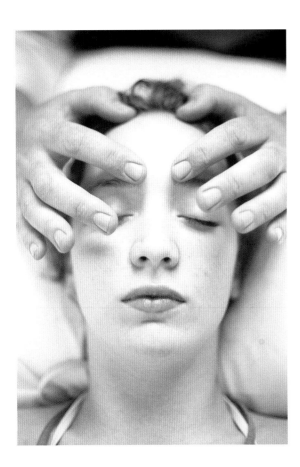
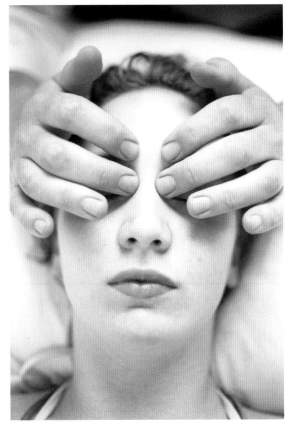

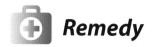 **Remedy**

Liver Cleanse

I have used a liver cleanse myself and with a number of clients to great effect. In fact it has been so successful in obviating the need for a gall bladder operation that one of my local doctors recently asked for the recipe to give to his clients. However, a word of warning – some cleanses can be very powerful and should only be done under the supervision of a naturopath or qualified nutritionalist. They should never be used in cases of serious conditions affecting the liver or gall bladder, when the person is feeling unwell or where there is the possibility of a gallstone becoming lodged.

There are many approaches to treating the liver – herbs such as Milk Thistle and drinks like fresh dandelion coffee can be very helpful on a regular basis. Dr Randolph Stone, the originator of Polarity Therapy, developed a number of liver and kidney cleanses which are described in his book *Health Building: The Conscious Art of Living Well*. One of the best cleanses is described in *The Amazing Liver Cleanse* by Andreas Moritz, available from St Ann's Press.

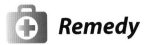

Remedy

Joints

Arthritic or Stiff Joints

A cupful of Epsom Salts added to the bath water will help to reduce stiffness. Epsom Salts can make the bath quite slippery and also be quite dehydrating, so it is advisable to have a bath mat and a glass of water nearby.

Swollen Joints

The following can help with swelling caused by injury to knees and ankles, etc. If the skin is sensitive it might be necessary to apply some Vaseline to the area first to protect it.

Grind down (if necessary) some pure washing soda (not Caustic Soda!) to the consistency of coarse salt. Place about 2-3 tablespoons of the dry soda in the middle of a cotton handkerchief and fold to make a small pack. Apply to the swollen area, hold in place with a bandage and cover with a hand towel or a disposable nappy. Leave the pack on for 6-8 hours overnight. If treating the knee, the pack is best applied just below the knee cap.

In the morning throw away the solidified crystals and repeat the process on alternate nights until the swelling reduces.

Bruising and Heat in Joints

This can be useful for treating inflammation in cases of tendonitis (for example tennis elbow). Soak some cotton wool in apple cider vinegar and dab on to the affected area every hour or so. You can also soak a bandage in cider vinegar and cover with cling film to prevent evaporation. It can be left on overnight, or for at least 4 -5 hours. You can advise the client to repeat daily until the heat subsides.

Left foot forward?

Bowen practitioners are generally advised to start working on the left side of the body first, particularly in the basic relaxation moves. Clinical experience has shown that starting on the right side will have less of an effect on regulating blood pressure than if you start on the left. Why is this?

Here are a few suggestions:

Lymph Flow

The way the lymphatic system works is that it is predominately left-sided. The majority of lymph in the body is collected via the thoracic (left lymphatic) duct, which receives lymph from the left side of the head, neck, chest, the left arm and the whole body below the ribs. Only lymph from the right arm, chest and right side of the head is collected by the right lymphatic duct.

Blood Flow

Apart from the fact that in the majority of people the heart is on the left, pressure in the left side of the heart is higher than the right side (around 120 mmHg in an adult in the left ventricle as opposed to 30 mmHg in the right ventricle). This is because the blood has to go all the way from the left side of your heart to your toes and still have enough pressure to bring the blood back to the right side of your heart. Simply speaking, the left side of the heart pumps blood around the body, while the right side of the heart pumps blood to the lungs.

Proteins

An intriguing question is why is it that almost all proteins in our body are built from L-amino acids (L stands for laevo- or left-handed). This question is studied in depth in Chris McManus's book *Right Hand, Left Hand*. He points out that 'Amino acids – the building blocks from which bodies are constructed – are left-handed, and any motor built from asymmetric components will turn in one particular direction.'

Muscle Fibres

There are different proportions of red and white muscle fibres on the left side of the body to the right. White fibres are called 'fast twitch', get easily fatigued and are needed for sports such as sprinting. Bowen work will therefore affect the left side of the musculature system differently to the right.

Mothers cradle babies on their left

According to Sieratzki and Wolf (*Sieratzki, J. S. & Woll, B. (1996), Why do mothers cradle babies on their left?* The Lancet):

- 80% of right and left handed mothers cradle babies on their left. Males no preference, but when males become fathers, 80% cradle left.

- In the left cradling position, maternal affective signals are given to the infants free left ear and processed by the right hemisphere, the hemisphere which is more advanced at this stage of development, and destined for the reception and processing of prosody.

- Left sided cradling facilitates the flow of auditory and visual communication between mother and infant and channels somato-affective feedback and infant sound to the mother's right hemisphere, which in turn tunes the melody of the mother's voice.

- Talmud: "A woman who begins to nurse her son should start on the left side, as the source of all understanding is from the left side." (Sefer Hassidim, 12th Century)

Best Foot Forward?

Why do we treat the better side first in many of the 'procedures'? It would appear that by treating the better side first:

- The body has a proprioceptive 'reference point' from which to self-adjust.
- It is less likely that the body will become overloaded, 'shut down' and not take on any more work.

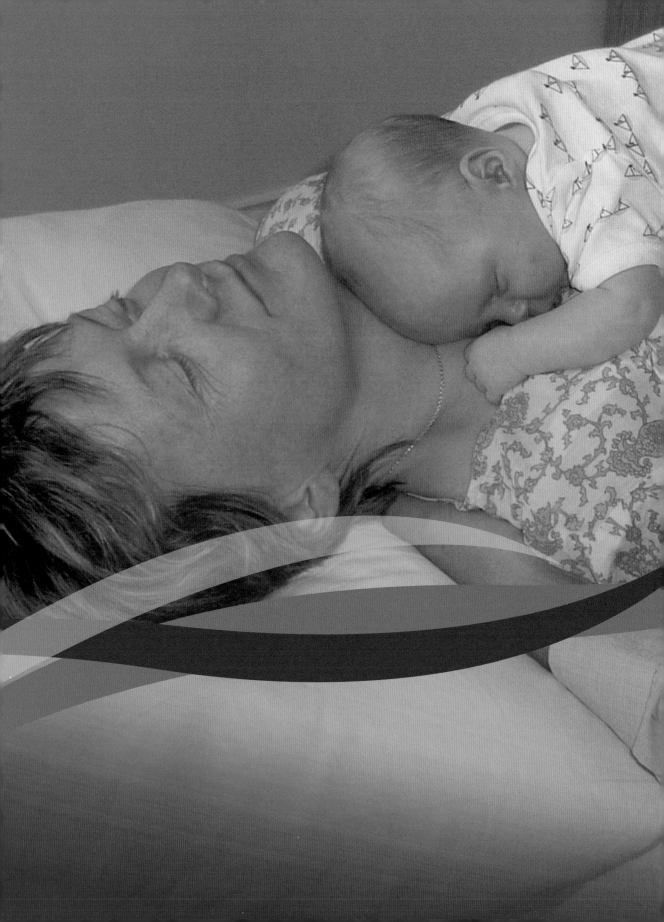

fertility & birth

Chapter 12

Assisting Conception

Lifestyle

There is plenty of evidence to suggest that just regular exercise for twenty minutes a day will increase a woman's chances of conceiving by around 50%. If you add to that certain dietary changes and drinking good quality water, these lifestyle changes are the most useful advice you can give a couple trying to conceive.

It is a good idea to get both partners involved so that they can support each other - the changes do not have to be rigorous. One of the best books on the subject is *Fit for Fertility,* by Michael Dooley, which is a mine of practical, easy to read information on the lifestyle changes that couples can do to improve their chances of conceiving.

For both partners regular exercise and eating a more alkaline diet will help (see appendix for a list of acid and alkaline-forming foods). Drinking more alkaline water (such as ionized water) can help in this process. 'Willow' water, available from many supermarkets, is fairly alkaline and also has traces of salicin which is reported to have anti-cancer properties.

One of the key things for both parties is to avoid endocrine disrupting chemicals found in pesticides, herbicides and some plastics. These can have a disastrous effect on sperm count and quality as many of them act as xeno-oestrogens or oestrogen mimicking molecules.

Many plastics and some cosmetics contain phthalates which, according to research by Prof Shanna Swan at the University of Rochester, New York, are associated with a lowering of sperm count. Phthalates are used in plastics to soften them so are found in higher densities in the soft plastics than in reusable polypropylene (PP) bottles used, for example, in cyclists' water bottles. This type of plastic is also used in water cooler bottles, baby bottles and many other uses. There is evidence that PP plastics leach bisphenol A, and that the leaching is worse when bleach is used on the plastic, a practice which many people use when their bottles get dirty.

Phthalates also tend to leach out into food – for example from the plastic lining in some canned foods, and most particularly

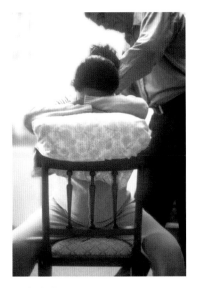

©John Wilks

from plastics into dairy products such as cheese and milk. Microwaving food, apart from changing its cellular structure, has a similar effect in terms of leaching phthalates from its plastic containers. In the USA and some other countries, many plastic bottles available in shops are marked as being either high or low in phthalates.

Research by Prof John Sumpter at Brunel University has also shown that the cocktails of chemicals (ie pesticides, herbicides, phalates, household products etc) found in tap water and food have a cumulative effect much stronger than when these chemicals are tested individually.

The best advice for a couple then, is to get on an organic diet, drink filtered or good quality bottled water and try and avoid dairy products, particularly those that have been in contact with plastic. Alcohol and smoking are an obvious no – no in this situation. The consumption of alcohol, particularly beer (it is very high in natural oestrogens), tends to lower sperm count.

If the above doesn't persuade them to make these changes, then a study published in the journal Endocrinology by Professor Ana Soto of Tufts University, Boston will. It shows that a mother's exposure to bisphenol A – a weak oestrogen mimic found in the plastic lining in food cans, alters the development of her child's mammary glands at the time of puberty and narrows the distance between the anus and the vagina, making a natural birth more difficult for her child.

Alarmingly, another study published in the journal Science by a team from Washington University has also showed that the effects of these endocrine disrupters pass down through generations and affect not only fertility in children and grand-children, but also their DNA.

Treatment Plans

It is a good idea wherever possible to treat both partners. You can do this in the same room as long as they can refrain from talking to each other and are able to relax.

One of the few contra-indications in Bowen work is performing the coccyx procedure on a woman during pregnancy. It is, therefore, important to ensure the client is not already pregnant. Suggest that she takes a pregnancy test if there is any doubt. The only situation one might consider doing the coccyx procedure during childbirth might be if the placenta fails to descend. It should not be used to speed up labour or bring it on, as a speedy delivery may be uncomfortable and potentially dangerous for both the mum and the baby.

One of the main criticisms some consultants have about complementary therapies and fertility is that it might delay the couple from seeking orthodox treatment until after it is too late; in other words, beyond the time a woman may be fertile. You might want to talk to the couple about this and make them aware of their choice in the matter.

Tom Bowen's conception protocol

When couples came to Tom Bowen for help with conception, he would always first 'balance' the body and address any postural issues in the normal way. He endeavoured to treat both partners as much as possible. Practitioners nowadays have adopted the protocol he developed with good success. However in many situations, doing the coccyx procedure on its own once or twice is enough.

Tom Bowen's recommended way of treating infertility was as follows:

- Address the coccyx from the side of pain (if there is one) and if one side is sensitive then address that side. If neither side is sensitive then address the left side.

- If in 3 consecutive sessions the coccyx shows sensitivity on the same side, then perfom the coccyx procedure from the opposite side in the next session. Continue with this pattern until a regular menstrual cycle is established.

- Treat the partner intermittently with whatever procedures are necessary to balance his body or alternately until the periods are regular.

- As close to the next period as possible perform the coccyx procedure only. Ask the couple to refrain from sex for 13 days after the treatment. Ideally, treat the partner with the Coccyx procedure at the same time.

- Make an appointment to see them in 2 month's time but ask the woman to take a pregnancy test before the next session in case she has conceived.

- If she isn't pregnant then you can repeat the coccyx procedure as above and see her again in 2 months.

IVF

The process of going through an assisted conception can be very stressful for both partners. Added to this, the strong medication that is used to alter patterns of ovulation can have a strong short-term effect on the woman's emotional health. She might become unusually angry, upset or depressed. Because of this it is inadvisable to stick rigidly to the above protocol. A better solution is to assist the couple through this difficult time by working simply and gently to reduce stress levels. This more than anything will make conception more likely.

Procedures such as the BRM's, the kidney, the TMJ and the pelvic all help in this process. The coccyx procedure would probably be unhelpful during this time, at least on the woman, as it can have such a strong effect on the hormonal system which will already have enough to do coping with the effects of the medication.

During Pregnancy

There is much to be said for treating a woman well before she gets pregnant. Bowen is so good at getting the body healthy on a cellular and tissue level that it can really help the body be more receptive. The downside of treating a woman who is pregnant (especially in the early stages) and who has never had a Bowen session before, is that it may produce a strong de-toxifying effect on the body. This might not be so good for the foetus if toxins pass through the placenta.

It has been noticed that Bowen work on pregnant horses who have never had a Bowen treatment before can result in spontaneous abortion. Although this has not been documented in humans, it would seem reasonable to suggest that if a mother-to-be has enjoyed a fairly toxic lifestyle (smoking, drinking, lack of exercise etc) before getting pregnant, her body will go into a natural 'detox' after a Bowen session which could be dangerous for the baby.

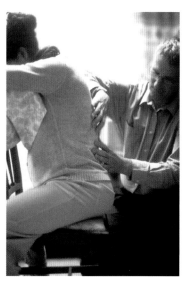

One way to avoid a toxic overload would be to start by doing very little on the first few sessions, making sure that they drink a lot of water, and avoid doing moves 3 & 4 of the neck until appropriate. It is highly inadvisable to work on pregnant mothers in the first trimester in any case because of the high risk of miscarriage.

Rick Minnery, a highly experienced midwife, has found that performing the pelvic and respiratory moves, much in the same way as for the work to address the psoas, can be effective in turning babies who are posterior (back to back) or breach. Acupuncture has been used to 'turn' babies or achieve optimal foetal positioning, but Bowen can also be effective.

The moves I usually do in these cases are:

BRM 1, moves 1 – 4
BRM 2, moves 1 – 4 (top stoppers) and moves 9 – 16
Kidney
Lower Respiratory moves 3 – 5
Pelvis

Bowen during Labour

Bowen has been used in labour wards and home births all over the world and can be very helpful in easing the potential discomfort of the delivery. Moves can be performed between each contraction and wherever it is needed (except for the coccyx procedure). Procedures such as the upper back, pelvis and sacrum have all been found to be helpful. As stated above, the coccyx procedure can be helpful to bring down the placenta after the baby has been delivered.

We shall discuss working with babies in the next chapter, suffice to say that I would not advise working on the baby within a few days of birth as there are so many important things that have to happen in terms of bonding and settling and one would not want to do anything that might get in the way. The only time I would suggest work on a baby less than a week after delivery would be if there is some problem such as the baby being born with the cord around its neck or having difficulty feeding or breathing. Obviously in these situations it is essential to work immediately.

Legal restrictions do apply in some countries in working with babies (for example in Sweden) and with mothers for a few days after birth (in the UK). It is always advisable to check with the mother's or the child's doctor or midwife and ask permission before working on them.

Work done by pre-natal and birth psychologists, such as Frank Lake, and experts on attachment theory like John Bowlby can be very helpful in understanding some of the strong imprinting that goes on during pregnancy and just after birth. More recently Sue Gerhardt has brought many elements of recent research and an understanding of bonding in her book *Why Love Matters: How Affection Shapes a Baby's Brain*. This book is highly recommended for all parents and potential parents.

Chapter *13*

Birth – First Impressions

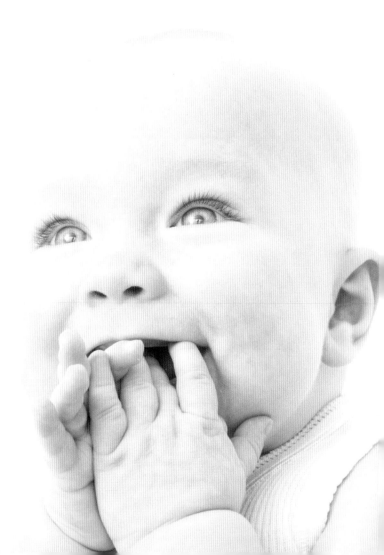

It is well documented that Tom Bowen would work on women in the later stages of pregnancy whenever they needed it. His view was that because the baby was moving around in the womb, it was similar to a re-injury. This justified breaking the 5 – 10 day rule between treatments.

We have talked about the need for caution during pregnancy – however certain procedures can really help open up the pelvic floor and greatly ease the process of childbirth. The pelvic, sacral, hamstrings and respiratory procedures will all have a highly beneficial effect.

The process of birth is a complex one and has many potential ramifications for the baby both on a physical and psychological level. Babies' nervous systems work far slower than adults and they tend to find anything that happens too fast distressing. Hence a fast delivery, although possibly easier for the mother, may not be such a good thing from the baby's point of view.

For this reason, it is a good idea to slow down ones movements and speech when treating babies, avoid any bright lights in the treatment room and have the temperature nice and warm.

Babies who have experienced a quick delivery can feel quite 'jangled'. They may be difficult to settle and may easily exhibit the Moro reflex (primitive startle reflex). Their sympathetic nervous system will often be over-activated and constantly on alert, making it difficult for them to feel comfortable and settled.

These kind of babies can be quite difficult to treat and in my experience will need a few sessions before they begin to feel more comfortable in themselves.

It is of course quite possible to perform any Bowen 'procedure' on a baby. The basic Bowen work for babies consists of the top stoppers and a variation on the lower respiratory work. For many babies this is enough to have a profound effect on their mood and well-being, as well as being highly beneficial for colicky babies.

With unsettled babies other work might help, such as the coccyx, the kidney or the TMJ procedure. As with animals, what is crucial is to gain their trust and not force anything on them against their will.

Babies have very clear body language and their comfort zone must be respected at all times. There is a very different quality to therapeutic touch as opposed to the loving touch of a parent, and a baby can feel your intention as you begin to make contact and intend to work in a particular area of their body. They will make it very clear by turning away, wriggling or even pushing you away if they are not happy with you working in a particular place.

Usually that area will be holding the tissue memory of some trauma related to birth. It is inadvisable, therefore, to work around a baby's head or neck on a first session. Babies usually 'hold' too much in this area for it to be safe for them.

Every type of birth will have its own dynamic to it and every baby will respond differently to that. Some babies have a highly resilient nature and can withstand the most terrible birth with apparently little consequence. For other babies the slightest upset will put their noses out of joint.

'Normal' Deliveries

Of course, as any mother will tell you, there is no such thing as a 'normal' birth. However, around 50% of births in the west are LOA or Left (side of the mum) Occiput (of the baby) Anterior (to the mum). This involves a fairly gentle rotation as the baby descends through the pelvic outlet.

There are all kinds of variants to vaginal deliveries, each with their own shorthand for describing them. In midwifery, the main landmarks are the baby's occiput (O), sacrum (S) and chin (M for mentum). For the mum, the landmarks are the mother's pelvis anterior (A ie the pubis), posterior (P) left (L) or right (R).

In a LOA birth the gentle rotation of the baby results in its face making contact with the mum's sacrum and coccyx, putting quite a degree of pressure on both. Then as the baby's head crowns, there is a rotation back to the side-on position. If left to nature,

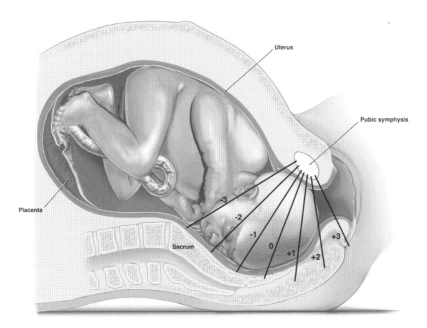

Left occiput anterior – the optimal foetal position for birth

the baby's posterior shoulder (its left shoulder in most cases) will be born first, though often in delivery rooms the anterior shoulder is birthed first. This often results in undue strain being placed on the brachial plexus area and it is not uncommon for babies' clavicles to be broken in this position (usually the right side).

A posterior birth (or 'back to back'), where the baby's back is towards the back of the mother, involves a 180 degree rotation down through the birth canal and might be described as OP.

Posterior births have ramifications for the baby's neck and jaw. As the baby becomes engaged in the rim of the mum's pelvis, the first thing it will experience is contact with the top of the mum's sacrum (the sacral promontory) and then the pubis. In a LOA position the baby will feel this on its parietal and temporal bones just above the ears as a compressive and dragging force down towards its feet. In an OP position the baby will feel it at the occiput and frontal bones.

During labour and with each contraction, the baby will assist by pushing hard with its legs. This is an important process for the baby and encourages mobilisation down through the lower part of its body.

For babies that have gone through a C-section delivery this mobilisation never happens and could be one reason why many are often slow to crawl or to walk. Bowen work on the lower part of the body for these babies can be highly beneficial.

Interventions

Treating babies can be much more complicated when interventions have been used at birth. The various possibilities are the use of pain-relieving drugs such as pethidine and epidurals and mechanical interventions like forceps, ventouse (vacuum extraction), caesarean and/or various types of foetal monitoring.

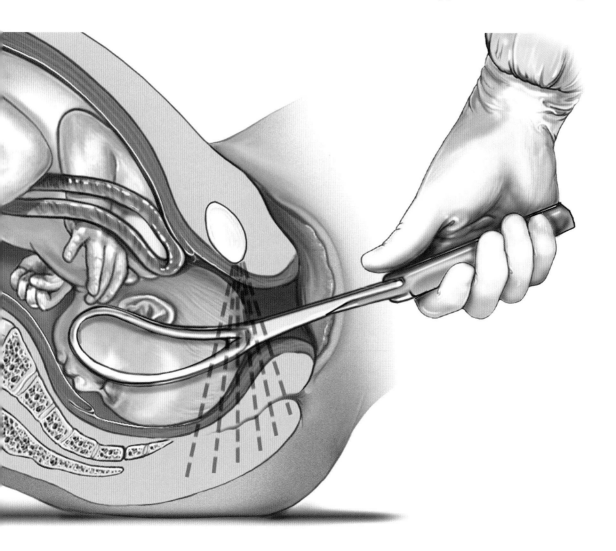

Forceps

Forceps need a lot of skill to be used safely as they put considerable medial compression around the temporal areas of the baby. Because various nerves around the temporal area are so vulnerable to compressive forces, great care has to be exercised. The nerves most affected by forceps are the vagus, (cranial nerve X), the spinal accessory (X1) and the glossopharangeal (1X). The effect of this might be to cause problems with digestion (eg colic or a sluggish digestive tract), hypertonus in the neck muscles, neck restriction (torticollis is quite common) or feeding problems.

The neck and TMJ work can be highly beneficial for babies born with forceps, although commonly they won't want you anywhere near their head and particularly their temporal area (around the ears) until levels of trust have been built up over a few sessions.

The baby's neck is not really designed for the strong pulling forces exerted on it with forceps (which can sometimes be extreme). Likewise with emergency Caesarian deliveries and suction, strong forces of traction and twisting can be fed into the baby's neck that can put a lot of strain on the short sensitive muscles and ligaments there. For this reason some gentle neck moves can be helpful in addressing issues there that may well manifest in symptoms such as colic and/or restlessness.

Suction, Vacuum Extraction and Ventouse

Ventouse deliveries are being used more and more these days, with about 10% of all births in the UK now being assisted with suction caps.

Vacuum extraction (as it is called in the USA) can of course be a life-saver for both mum and baby, but it does have ramifications, particularly for the baby. Firstly it is a very strong local pressure to the back of the baby's head (usually the occiput), which is very uncomfortable even for adults to experience. For the baby, birth is the first really strong imprinting of physical sensation that goes on and if one thinks about the whole phenomenon of tissue memory, then ventouse is potentially an extremely strong imprinting on a tissue level, along with its associated emotional imprinting.

One of the reasons given for using ventouse over forceps is that there is much less potential for intra-cranial pressure with ventouse. However, this doesn't account for the fact that ventouse exerts an extraordinary amount of pressure locally which has much more potential for distortion patterns to be fed into the baby's cranium. Usually it is not just a question of attaching the cap and pulling straight down in line with the birth canal. Often the midwife or obstetrician has to pull off centre to bring the baby down.

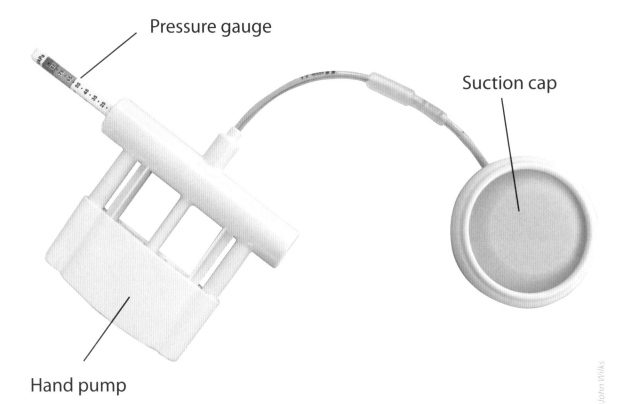

Pressure gauge

Suction cap

Hand pump

©John Wilks

Because the baby's occiput is not fused at birth there is potential for distortion patterns to be fed into the base of the occiput around the condyles which will then affect the occipito-atlanteal joint (the O/A junction) and the ventricles, particularly the fourth ventricle. Ventricles are the fluid filled spaces in the brain and what tends to happen is that the fourth ventricle that goes down towards the brain stem can get pulled up along with the spinal cord towards the foramen magnum.

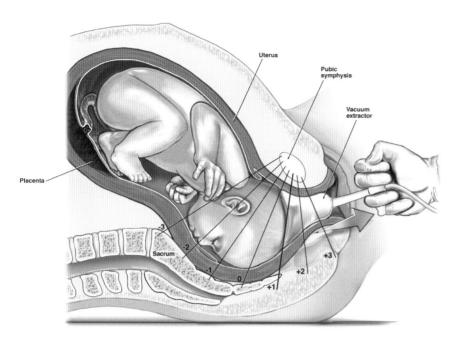

The major issue with Ventouse is the potential for distortion at the condyles and around the temporal area which then has a direct effect on the TMJ, the hard palate and the bite. From what we have seen earlier this can have implications for postural issues later on as well as affecting some of the major cranial nerves, including the Vagus.

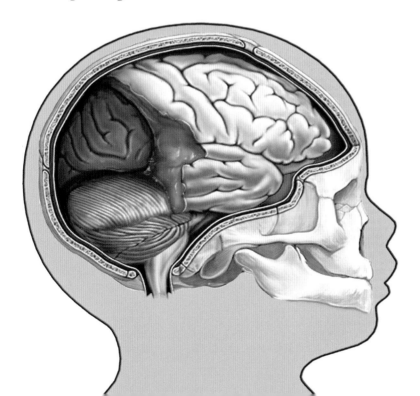

Assessing Babies

Babies instinctively know when help is at hand and will usually show you clearly where they need attention. They will also show you when they do not want to be touched in a particular area by moving away or turning their head. Tom Bowen used to examine the sclera (the whites) of the eyes in babies who were over 3 months old to see if they had a neck restriction. One of the reasons for this may be that the vertebral artery, which supplies some of the blood to the brain, comes up through foramina in the cervical vertebrae and then does a complicated loop around the base of the occiput before entering the cranium. A restriction in blood supply (which could manifest itself as blueness in the sclera) would result from a neck restriction on either side.

If a baby has a neck restriction it is common for it to prefer to have its head to one side rather than the other. A mother will have noticed this and one can test it by getting the baby to follow the movement of your finger with its eyes. Babies are naturally inquisitive and will follow any movement with their gaze. You may notice as you bring your finger round that there is some resistance to following your finger. You can ask the mother if they notice that their baby prefers to feed off one breast rather than the other. This can also be indicative of a neck restriction.

An easy way to assess whether or not babies may need the top of their neck attending to is to feel around the back of their heads close to where we do moves 3 & 4 – in other words around the occipital crest. You may find (especially in babies who have had a ventouse delivery) that one side is more anterior to the other or that some distortion is held there.

One can also assess by looking down from the top of the baby's head. If you look at the position of the ears you may notice that one is anterior to the other. Again, this is not uncommon with ventouse babies and will indicate that you need to address the TMJ area.

Ventouse has only been used fairly recently (from the 1970's onwards), so it is probable that Tom Bowen didn't come across it in his practice. However, it is essential to address it (ie the problem) with the whole neck procedure (rather than just moves

5 & 6) because it affects the whole cranium and particularly the attachments of the trapezius at the back of the head.

Umbilical Shock

One of the reasons that work around the diaphragm may be so helpful for babies is that it helps to address the issue of umbilical shock (or umbilical effect, as it is termed by psychologists).

A lot has to happen very quickly right after the baby is born. Firstly, it has to go from getting oxygen from the mother to using its lungs for the first time. This involves a small valve in the heart closing over (the foramen ovale) within a few minutes. There also have to be rapid changes in the liver and the bladder at the same time.

If the umbilical cord is cut before it stops pulsating then these changes have to happen even quicker and the body is forced into an unnatural situation. Many therapists believe that this may be a reason for conditions such as 'hole in the heart' and bladder and liver complications later in life. One of the sad consequences of stem cell research has been that parents want to store umbilical blood as a kind of 'health insurance' for their children. Unfortunately this involves taking blood from the umbilicus immediately the baby is born, neccessitating a premature cutting of the cord.

Primitive Reflexes

There are a whole host of reflexes that the foetus begins to display in the womb just a few weeks after conception. These reflexes have a certain life-cycle before they get replaced by more complex reflexes after birth.

Some of the more well known primitive reflexes are:

• The Moro (or startle) reflex which emerges around 9 weeks in utero and gets inhibited at anywhere between two to six months of life.

• The Asymetrical Tonic Neck Reflex (ATNR) which emerges

around 4 months in utero and is inhibited at around 5 months after birth. This causes the arms to bend and the legs to extend when the head is in flexion and the arms to extend and the legs to flex when the head is extended.

The Moro or startle reflex

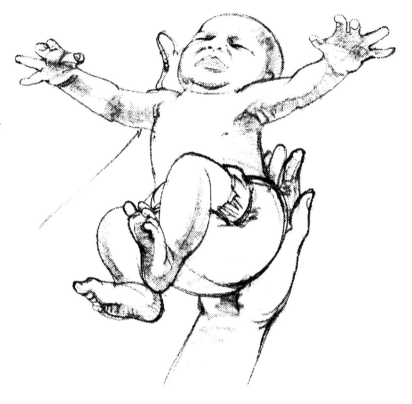

Image reproduced with kind permission of the author from Goddard SA, 1996 A teacher's window into the child's mind. Fern Ridge Press. Eugene. OR and Goddard SA, 2001 Reflexes, learning and behavior. Fern Ridge Press. Eugene. OR.

- The Spinal Galant which emerges around the time of the Moro reflex but usually inhibits a bit later.

- The sucking and rooting reflex which starts around 4 months in utero and inhibits at around 4 months after birth.

- The Babinski reflex which starts at birth and inhibits anywhere up to 2 years.

What is interesting to note in babies is how certain reflexes may be over or under-active or fail to inhibit. The Moro reflex, which involves the baby's arms going backwards when there is a possibility it might be dropped or it is exposed to loud noise, is a primitive startle reflex. It involves a sudden strong activation of the sympathetic nervous system and a generally hyper-aroused state. The second part to this reflex, where the system calms down and the parasympathetic system becomes more evident, is a closing of the arms over the chest. Often in babies who have had traumatic births or, in particular, Caesarian deliveries, the first part of this reflex will be dominant and express itself frequently at the slightest upset. Sometimes such babies even exhibit it just as they are dropping off to sleep, as though being off guard is felt as dangerous for them.

What an over-expressed Moro reflex will tell us is that the baby's sympathetic nervous system is generally over-active and it would probably be helpful for it if we could work to dissipate some of that held charge by working the kidneys, respiratory, coccyx or TMJ.

Experts who work with primitive reflexes use clever exercises to encourage reflexes to inhibit and be replaced by more complex and refined reflexes such as the adult startle reflex. Children who fidget a lot often have certain primitive reflexes that have failed to inhibit. Others can have an effect on a child's development.

Tom Bowen was probably aware of the Spinal Galant reflex when he developed the bedwetting procedure. This reflex occurs when you stimulate the erector spinae muscles by stroking down the back. The baby will flex the leg and urinate. It could be that using our extra holding points and doing the coccyx procedure helps to inhibit this reflex in children where it hasn't been replaced by more complex control centres.

More information on primitive reflexes and how they affect child development can be found in the book *Reflexes, Learning and Behaviour – a window into the child's mind,* by Sally Goddard.

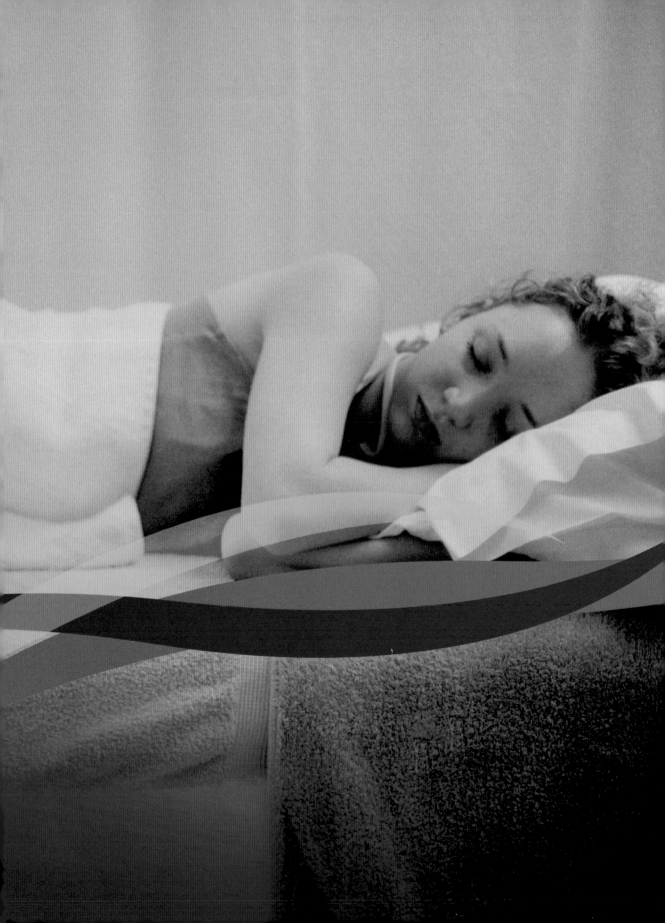

life after treatment

Chapter 14

What goes in must come out

Tom Bowen was intensely interested in nutritional and naturopathic approaches to health at a time in Australia when it wasn't fashionable to be so. These days it is more common for complementary therapists to pay much more attention to nutrition, even though most medical schools only spend a few hours on the subject in their medical degree courses.

The issue of acid and alkalinity is a hot topic when it comes to a discussion about health, particularly in relation to diseases like cancer and arthritis. Many self-help books on the subject advise a more alkaline diet for arthritis and an avoidance of the nightshade family of vegetables – potatoes, aubergines and tomatoes, for example.

The chart shown below is distilled from a variety of books and is by no means complete or authoritative. There are some good books out on the subject, particularly the series *The pH Miracle,* by Robert and Shelley Young. There are also websites which debate the merits of a more alkaline diet. If you do a Google search for 'acid alkaline diet' some good charts will come up, although many have contradictory information.

Part of the confusion has been around the fact that many writers try to equate alkalinity with a more yang diet and acid with a more yin diet. The concept of yin and yang foods comes from Macrobiotics and its proponent in the West, Michio Kuchi, and stems from a very different understanding of the effects of food on the body in addition to a purely biological one. One book that explores this approach is *Acid and Alkaline*, by Herman Aihara.

What is important to understand is that alkalinity is dependent on how one's body metabolises food. In other words, lemons (which are essentially acid in nature) are metabolised by the body into alkalising food and have an alkalising effect generally on the tissues.

Tom Bowen was keen to promote a more alkaline diet for a wide range of conditions. For example, he would suggest that children who are wetting the bed go on an 80% alkaline to 20% acid-forming diet. As a general rule, foods like red meat, refined foods and drinks are acid forming.

An interesting feature of today's lifestyle is that stress tends to create acidity in the body. Research has shown that negative thoughts create by far the strongest effect in terms of making the system more acid than almost any food. Positive thinking, love and laughter will create a more alkaline body.

Water

These days our tap water is quite acidic unless you are lucky enough to live in an area which is supplied with good quality spring water. Water quality and type is a hotly debated subject these days, with most 'experts' offering conflicting opinions on the subject. One of the most comprehensive sources of information (although not necessarily impartial!) can be found at *www.cyber-nook.com/water/index.html*.

There are, however, some well-researched conclusions when it comes to what kind of water we should be drinking:

• Tap water is acidic and contains many substances that are harmful to health including (in some areas of the world) fluoride, heavy metals, chlorine and residues of prescribed and non-prescribed medication. It is estimated that the majority of the UK population is now imbibing significant levels of anti-depressants and the contraceptive pill in its drinking water.

• Distilled water that Tom Bowen used to advise if a patient was undergoing a reaction, or if their system generally was toxic, is also quite acidic, and should not be recommended long term as it is denuded of essential trace minerals.

• De-ionised water is quite alkaline. A water ioniser or de-ioniser produces 2 streams of water – one acid (which you can use to wash in and water your household plants) and the other alkaline. Some commentators, however, have pointed out that the ionised stream is high in calcium which may not be so good for your arteries.

An interesting area of research is how water molecules group in different types of water. In de-ionised water, for example, they are arranged in smaller groups and this allows an easier passage through the cell membranes of the body. This may account for why some patients with conditions such as ME and fibromyalgia have found drinking such water helpful.

There are many excellent water filters and filtration systems on the market. Two of the best are made by the Pure H2O Company (www.pureh2o.co.uk) and the PiMag system made by Nikken (www.nikken.com). One of the most visionary researchers on the subtle qualities of water was the Austrian scientist Viktor Schauberger (1885 – 1958), whose concept of water as a living organism has profound implications for us today.

Testing your pH levels

PH levels in one's body change throughout the day but the normal range is something like this:

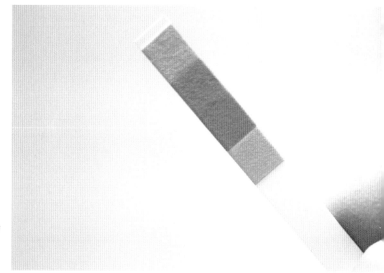

- Saliva pH 6.8 - 7.8
- Urine pH 6.3 - 7.2

You can determine the body's pH through self-testing urine and saliva with pH/litmus paper. It can be helpful to test yourself daily or weekly to see how your pH levels fluctuate.

If you are testing saliva, it is important to realise that alkaline levels will be greater after meals because there is an abundance of alkaline-rich minerals in saliva.

If you are testing urine, you will probably find that in the morning and during fasting there will be more acid waste. You should see your urine pH become more alkaline as the day progresses.

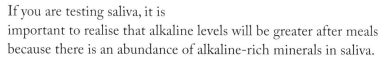

The chart below has been compiled from several sources and is by no means complete or authoritative.

Acid – Alkaline Food Chart

Tom Bowen advocated a balanced 80/20 diet for many of his clients, composed of 80% alkaline forming foods and 20% acid forming foods.

ALKALIZING FOODS

VEGETABLES
Garlic, Watercress, Beans (green, lima, string, sprouts), Beets, Broccoli, Cabbage, Carrot, Cauliflower, Celery, Chard, Chicory, Chives, Cowslip, Cucumber, Dandelions, Dill, Dock, green, Dulse, seaweed, Endive, Edible Flowers, Eggplant / Aubergine, Kale, Lettuce, Mushrooms (most), Mustard Greens, Parsnips (high glycemic), Peas, Peppers, Potatoes, Pumpkin, Sorrel, Spinach, Spring greens, Squash, Turnips and tops, Alfalfa, Barley Grass, Wheat Grass, Wild Greens

FRUITS
Apple, Apricot, Avocado, Cantaloupe, Carob (pod only), Cherries, Currants, Dates/Figs, Grapes, Honeydew Melon, Mangoes, Papayas, Peach, Pear, Raisins, All Berries, Watermelon

PROTEIN
Eggs, Whey Protein Powder, Cottage Cheese, Goats Milk, Yogurt, Almonds, Chestnuts, Tofu (fermented), Flax Seeds, Pumpkin Seeds, Squash Seeds, Sunflower Seeds, Millet, Sprouted Seeds, Nuts

OTHER
Apple Cider Vinegar, Bee Pollen, Lecithin Granules, Probiotic Cultures, Green Juices, Veggies Juices, Fresh Fruit Juice, Mineral Water, Alkaline Antioxidant Water, Green Tea, Herbal Tea, Dandelion Tea, Ginseng Tea, Banchi Tea, Kombucha

SWEETENERS
Stevia

SPICES/SEASONINGS
Cinnamon, Curry, Ginger, Mustard, Chili Pepper, Sea Salt, Miso, Tamari, All Herbs

CITRUS FRUITS
Citrus fruits are acidic, yet because of their high calcium content they produce an alkaline effect during the digestive process. People can experience citrus fruits as alkaline or as acidic.

ACIDIFYING FOODS

FATS & OILS
Avocado Oil, Canola Oil, Corn Oil, Hemp Seed Oil, Flax Oil, Lard, Olive Oil, Safflower Oil, Sesame Oil, Sunflower Oil

FRUITS
Cranberries, Chestnuts (roasted), All preserves, jellies & jams (canned, sugared, glazed fruits), Bananas (green), Plums, Prunes & prune juice, Olives & all pickles

GRAINS
All flour products, Rice Cakes, Amaranth, Barley, Buckwheat, Breads (all kinds), Corn, cornmeal, cornflakes, corn flour, Oats (rolled), Quinoi, Rice (all), Rye, Spelt, Kamut, Wheat, Hemp Seed

DAIRY
Cheese, Cow, Cheese, Goat, Cheese, Sheep, Butter, Cream, ice cream, Custard, Chocolate

NUTS & BUTTERS
Cashews, Brazil Nuts, Peanuts, Peanut Butter, Pecans, Tahini, Walnuts

ANIMAL PROTEIN
Beef, Carp, Clam, Chicken, Fish, Lamb, Lobster, Mussels, Oyster, Pork, Rabbit, Salmon, Shrimp, Scallops, Tuna, Turkey, Venison, Gelatine, Gravies

PASTA (WHITE)
Noodles, Macaroni, Spaghetti

OTHER
Distilled Vinegar, Wheat Germ, Cocoa, Coffee, Condiments, Dressings, Sauces, Eggs (esp. whites), Soda water, Tobacco

DRUGS & CHEMICALS
Chemicals, Drugs, Medicinal Drugs, Psychedelic, Pesticides, Herbicides

ALCOHOL
Beer, Spirits, Hard Liquor, Wine

BEANS & LEGUMES
Black Beans, Chick Peas, Green Peas, Kidney Beans, Lentils, Lima Beans, Pinto Beans, Red Beans, Soy Milk, White Beans, Rice Milk, Almond Milk

OTHER VEGETABLES
Brussel sprouts, Rhubarb, Tomato

ALKALIZERS
Cold showers, Love, Laughter, Hugs, Fresh air

ACIDIFIERS
Lack of sleep, Overwork, Worry, Tension, Anger, Jealousy, Resentment

Below are tables of common foods with an approximate potential
acidity or alkalinity, as present in one ounce of food.

Alkali-Forming Foods

Figs	30.0	Potatoes	2.0
Soy Beans	12.0	Pineapple	2.0
Lima Beans	12.0	Cabbage	1.8
Apricots	9.5	Grapefruit	1.7
Spinach	8.0	Tomatoes	1.7
Turnip/Beet tops	8.0	Peaches	1.5
Raisins	7.0	Apples	1.0
Almonds	3.6	Grapes	1.0
Carrots	3.5	Bananas	1.0
Dates	3.0	Watermelon	1.0
Celery	2.5	Millet	0.5
Cucumber	2.5	Brazil nuts	0.5
Cantaloupe	2.5	Coconuts	0.5
Lettuce	2.2	Buckwheat	0.5
Watercress	2.0		

Neutral (near/neutral) Foods

Milk		Vegetable oils
Butter		White sugar

Acid-Forming Foods

Oysters	5.0	Rice	2.5
Veal	3.5	W.Wheat/Rye bread	2.5
Most Fish	3.5	Most nuts (X-almond/brazil nut)	2.0
Organ meats	3.0	Natural Cheese	1.5
Liver	3.0	Lentils	1.5
Chicken	3.0	Peanuts	1.0
Fowl	3.0	Eggs	3.0
Most Grains	3.0		

Chapter 15

Being Professional

Research

One of the simplest and most cost-effective ways of validating one's work is to keep a client-centred record of treatments and their outcomes. There is an existing protocol which has been used by the British Acupuncture Council and the College of Homeopaths for many years and has been adopted by the Bowen Association in the UK. The original protocol was designed by Dr Charlotte Paterson in the South-West of England and provides an excellent method of validating data from a wide range of conditions.

The protocol is called MYMOP, which stands for Measure Your Medical Outcome Profile, and is shown below. This protocol and instructions can be photocopied for free. I have used this personally for many years with clients at my clinic in Dorset.

For a full list of published research on the Bowen Technique please see the appendix at the back of the book.

How to use MYMOP

Give copies of the forms to your clients and explain how to fill them in. Give clients the follow up forms to fill in a minimum of three times, preferably at weekly intervals. It is fine to carry on for longer if you feel like it - use your own assessment as to whether or not a longer follow-up period will be useful.

Young children and babies obviously cannot fill the forms out by themselves, so their carer can fill it out. It is essential that it is always the same person who fills out all the forms. It is suggested that the carer fills out the forms for children and babies up to five years of age. Between the ages of five and ten, the child can play an active part in filling in the form. From ten years, a child may like to fill out their own form, but this will no doubt vary from child to child.

A client can start filling out a follow-up form at any point during the course of treatment, however this must only be from that moment on, ie forms cannot be filled in retrospectively. It is fine for a client to refer to a condition diagnosed by a doctor even if the patient does not fully understand the diagnosis, but the patient should use their own terminology to describe their condition if they prefer.

It is easier to do the survey at the end of a session when hopefully there will tend to be a greater clarity about symptoms.

BOWTECH
The Bowen Association of the UK
MYMOP2

Full name... Date of birth....................................

Address and postcode...
Todays date.......................... Practitioner seen...

Choose one or two symptoms (physical or mental) which bother you the most. Write them on the lines Now consider how bad each symptom is, over the last week, and score it by circling your chosen number.

SYMPTOM 1:   0   1   2   3   4   5   6
.... As good as   As bad as
.... it could be   it could be

SYMPTOM 2:   0   1   2   3   4   5   6
.... As good as   As bad as
.... it could be   it could be

Now choose one activity (physical, social or mental) that is important to you, and that your problem makes difficult or prevents you doing. Score how bad it has been in the last week.

ACTIVITY: 0   1   2   3   4   5   6
.... As good as   As bad as
.... it could be   it could be

Lastly, how would you rate your general feeling of wellbeing during the last week?

0   1   2   3   4   5   6
As good as   As bad as
it could be   it could be

How long have you had your SYMPTOM 1, either all the time or on and off?
Less than 2 weeks ☐   2-4 weeks ☐   4-12 weeks ☐
3 months- 1 year ☐   Over 1 year ☐

Tick the box which best describes how you feel:

Cutting down or avoiding medication
is not important to me ☐
is a bit important to me ☐
is very important to me ☐

If you have answered that cutting down or avoiding medication **IS** important to you, write down what medication you would like to cut down or avoid, and how much of it you are taking at the moment.

BOWTECH
The Bowen Association of the UK
MYMOP2 follow-up

Full name.. Today's date.......................................

Please circle the number to show how severe your problem has been IN THE LAST WEEK
This should be YOUR opinion, no-one else's!

SYMPTOM 1:   0   1   2   3   4   5   6
.... As good as   As bad as
.... it could be   it could be

SYMPTOM 2:   0   1   2   3   4   5   6
.... As good as   As bad as
.... it could be   it could be

ACTIVITY: 0   1   2   3   4   5   6
.... As good as   As bad as
.... it could be   it could be

WELLBEING: How would   0   1   2   3   4   5   6
you rate your general   As good as   As bad as
feeling of wellbeing?   it could be   it could be

If an important new symptom has appeared please describe it and mark how bad it is below. Otherwise do not use this line.

SYMPTOM 3:   0   1   2   3   4   5   6
.... As good as   As bad as
.... it could be   it could be

The treatment you are receiving may not be the only thing affecting your problem. If there is anything else that you think is important, such as changes you have made yourself, or other things happening in your life, please write it here (write overleaf if you need more space):

If cutting down or avoiding medication is important to you , tick the box to show how this has changed since your previous MYMOP form:

Not much change ☐
Taking less medication ☐
Taking more medication ☐

Contact Their Doctor

One of the complaints many healthcare practitioners, including doctors, have is the lack of communication between practitioners responsible for their clients' care.

One of the simplest ways of promoting yourself and ensuring communication is to contact the client's doctor and inform them that they are coming to you for treatment. The way of doing this is described in the section on promoting yourself.

Creating a dialogue with other health professionals is highly effective in promoting good relations between doctor, client and practitioner, and will lead to a much more integrated and 'joined-up' approach to your clients' treatment. It is also an excellent way of promoting yourself as a practitioner.

It is important that if you have concerns about the person's response to the treatment, any deterioration in their condition or the advice/treatment they are receiving, then it is your responsibility to inform the doctor of your concerns. Again, this should only be done with the patient's written consent.

Notifiable Diseases

In the UK, there are a number of notifiable diseases that under the *Public Health (Infectious Diseases) Regulations Act 1988* you are obliged to inform The Health Protection Agency about. These diseases are listed on the *www.hpa.org.uk* website and include:

- Acute encephalitis
- Food poisoning
- Measles
- Meningitis
- Mumps
- Relapsing fever
- Rubella
- Tuberculosis
- Viral hepatitis (A, B and C)
- Whooping cough

The above list is not exhaustive. For a complete list please see the

HPA's website.

Record Keeping

In a court of law, if you have no records you have no defence. Therefore, the general advice on this is to always keep detailed case notes (bearing in mind that the client will always have the right to see them) and never throw them away.

Lawyers will advise that clients have a period of seven years after a treatment to make a claim against a practitioner. However, in some cases this has been extended under exceptional circumstances (eg in cases of abuse). Also this rule only comes into effect when a client turns 18. It is theoretically possible, therefore, that a client who you treated as a 3 month old child could turn around at age 25 and decide that he/she had been severely traumatised by the experience. An unlikely occurrence, but it is always better to be safe than sorry.

Confidentiality

Patient records should always be kept confidential and in a safe and secure place (preferably locked). There does, nonetheless, arise certain circumstances where patient confidentiality is over-ridden by concerns for the safety of others, particularly children. This might happen if, for example, you suspect that a child is being abused by an adult. The first thing in such a case is to get advice from your insurers or your professional association on how to proceed, as such situations can be a minefield.

A useful publication from the British Medical Association, *Doctors' Responsibilities in Child Protection Cases,* outlines one's responsibility in this regard and also lists recommendations from the General Medical Council. The Association's recent publication *The Right to Health: a Toolkit for Health Professionals,* also provides an excellent overview of the responsibilities of all healthcare practitioners. Both documents are available to download free from their website at *www.bma.org.uk*

Difficult Clients

We all have them – some more difficult than others. Sometimes things are said or done inadvertently during a consultation which might be misconstrued by either side.

It is obviously better if misunderstandings can be sorted out at the time and in such cases it is absolutely essential that a full record is made on the same day of the consultation – what was said or done and what the outcome was.

This report can then either be lodged with the clinic manager, or, if you are working from home, with your professional association. Most insurance companies also offer a free legal advice and mediation service should you need it.

Chapter 16

Promote yourself!

There is very little point in being the best therapist in the world if no-one knows about you. Promoting yourself does not necessarily mean being pushy or having to stand up in front of a hundred people and give a talk. There are simple and enjoyable ways of getting the word out there and the best way of all is to get your patients to do it for you. Do a good job and they will spread the word. To this end some of the best people to treat are hairdressers as most have bad backs and all have a captive audience.

Write to their doctors

One thing we have done in our clinic for many years is to write to the client's doctor to notify them that they are coming for treatment. On the clients medical questionnaire is a tick box which asks; 'Do we have your permission to write to your doctor and inform them that you are receiving treatment with the Bowen technique?' The vast majority of clients agree.

We then send a simple letter on clinic letterhead which goes something like this:

Dear Dr X

Mrs Doris Smith DOB 15.07.65

The above patient is coming to see me for treatment with the Bowen Technique.

If you have any questions about the treatment please phone me on the above number. I am at the clinic on Mondays and Thursdays from 9.30 to 6.00.

I enclose a leaflet for your information.

Yours sincerely

John Wilks, BTAA

This has the double advantage of opening up professional communication with your local doctors as well as the likelihood that at some stage your client's doctor will ask them how they are responding to your treatment. I have had a number of referrals as a result.

It also means that if you have concerns about your client at any stage (maybe they are not responding to treatment in the way you might expect or they have symptoms which are unusual and you feel need investigating) then you have already started a dialogue with their primary carer and it is easier to then contact them – always though with the client's permission.

Give talks

Giving talks need not be nerve-wracking, especially if you do it with a fellow practitioner. Groups such as the Women's Institute in the UK, Rotary clubs and special interest groups are always on the lookout for entertaining speakers. Usually the best idea is to keep it light, give plenty of heart-warming examples (case studies – but be sure to ask permission or change any personal details) and talk about yourself. When I was doing a lot of talks to the WI I used to break the ice by talking to them about the hazards of wearing bras - much to their amusement. Most audiences are not interested in too much technical detail – they like to hear your story – how you got into doing what you do. Best to spice it up with some demonstration and possibly talk about other related things like diet, water, exercise, ergonomics or whatever you feel comfortable with. By the time you've taken questions and judged the cake competition, an hour will have flown by. Most Women's Institutes will pay your travel expenses and give you a small fee and you are likely to come home with some delicious jam.

Offer free 20 minute appointments

Once someone has met you and they have received a taste of a Bowen session they will usually come back for more. I used to offer free taster sessions from time to time if I needed to boost my numbers and the take-up rate was always in excess of 50%. The best thing is to address their area of concern there and then either seated or, if there is time, lying on the couch.

You can set aside a morning for taster sessions – that way you can fit in 12 people in a morning. I guarantee that you will end up with at least 6 new clients out of it.

The way I used to promote these was to design a small A5 or A6 flier (postcard size) which said something like this:

Bad Back?

Frozen Shoulder?

Migraine Headaches?

Have you tried the Bowen Technique?

Free 20 minute taster sessions available on Tuesdays at the Homeville Bowen Clinic

Phone 01234 56789

You can display these on notice boards or you can ask your local health food store to pop one of the cards in each shopping bag for you.

Write articles

Your local paper is always looking for a story or sometimes for someone to write a regular health column. Always make sure that if you write about any case histories you have that client's express permission. Writing articles is not easy and needs a certain art to get the style right. If you have a friendly journalist friend, ask them how to do it.

Run open days

Open days at your local clinic are a good way of promoting the whole clinic. Best to have them on market days or Saturday mornings. Offer free teas and coffees or some other incentive to step inside.

There are many good books on promoting yourself and some useful ones written especially for complementary therapists. Two of the best are *How to Be a Successful Therapist*, by Celia Johnson and *Marketing for Complementary Therapists: 101 Tried and Tested Ways to Attract Clients*, by Steven Harold.

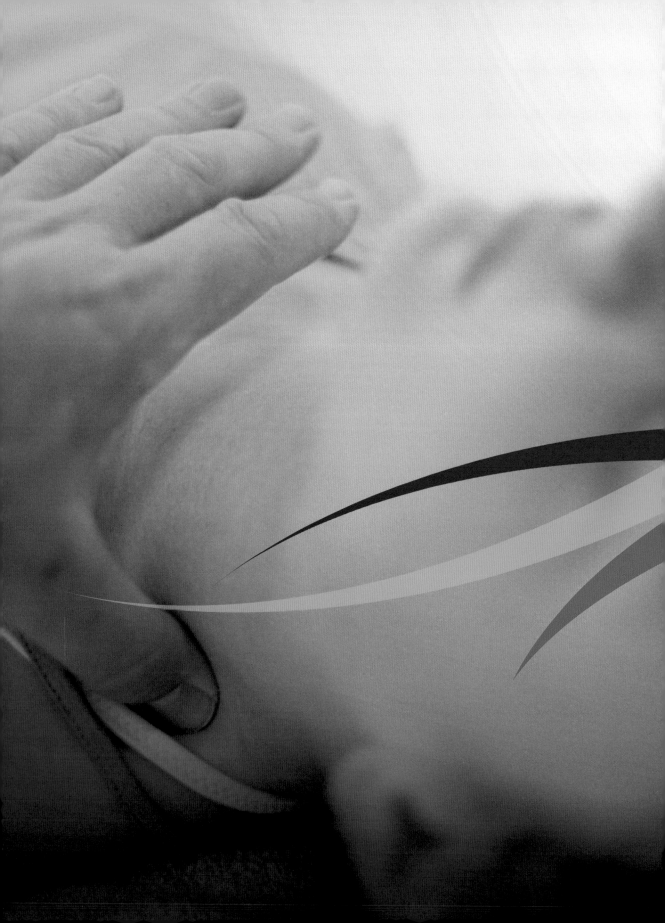

the therapeutic relationship

by su fox

Chapter 17

Introduction: Therapeutic Relationship Vignettes

First Scenario

Imagine – or remember, because this may have been your own experience once upon a time – that you're arriving for your first Bowen technique session. You don't know anything about this, in fact you've never visited any sort of complementary therapist before, but a friend of a friend recommended it for back pain. And you've had back pain for as long as you can remember, and had got to the point of thinking that you'd have to just put up with it because all the tests that the doctor sent you for could find no cause. You're feeling apprehensive, but also a little bit hopeful. You arrive at the clinic early, not wanting to be late for your 10 o'clock appointment, and the receptionist smiles, asks you to take a seat and says 'Tim's expecting you, he won't be long.'

At 10 o'clock exactly, Tim comes to the reception, walks over to you smiling and asks, 'Hello. You must be (fill in your own name). Come with me.' And leads you into a treatment room. There's a couch, like the one at the doctors, and two chairs by the table. You notice there isn't a computer. Tim asks you to sit down. 'What brings you here today?' he says. You explain about your back problem. He asks you to show him exactly where you feel the pain; and whether it's worse at certain times of day, or when you do certain activities. He makes notes as you talk, but looks at you, and you get the feeling that he is really interested. You tell him about all the medical tests and he asks for dates, and the name of the consultant and the hospital. Then he says 'I'm just going to ask a few questions about your general health, to see if there are any other things to take into account when working with you. After this, he asks what you already do to help your back pain, which surprises and pleases you, because it's as if he's thinking that this is a collaborative effort. He's giving you credit for the fact that you have been living with this condition for a long time and, therefore, know more about what it's like than he does. He also enquires, and this one really stumps you, why you think you might have back pain, what the meaning is for you. You find yourself thinking about this question over the next few days.

Tim puts his notes on the table and asks if you know anything about the Bowen technique. 'No' you reply 'except a friend of a friend said it works.' 'That's right' says Tim, 'it can, especially for the back pain of the kind that I think you've got. Let me tell you about it'. And he fills you in a little; about the Australian called Tom Bowen who started it, and how it works gently, with different layers of tissue in the body to release old stuck patterns. 'In a moment I'll ask you to take off your shoes and jacket and lie down. If you're cold, I've got the blanket there to cover you up. I'll make gentle contact with some muscles on your back and do some light moves. And then I'll go out of the room. I know this might seem a bit strange, but the reason is to leave your body completely alone to readjust to the moves I've made. Then I'll come back in and perhaps do another few moves.

You may or may not feel much during the treatment, but this is a powerful treatment. Most people feel very relaxed during the treatment, so if you feel like going to sleep that's fine. When we finish I'll go through what to expect with you. But I would ask you not to have any other sort of treatment in the next week. You said your physiotherapy had stopped anyway? Good, because other treatments could possibly interfere with the effect of the Bowen. And I'd recommend that you have three or four sessions with me, we can make the appointments later, and we'll see then how your back's doing. And I know we talked about this on the phone, but each session costs £30, and you can pay me at the end each time before you go. Do you understand? Is all that ok with you? Anything that wasn't clear? You're nodding yes to his questions, then remember you've got a dentist's appointment on Friday, and wonder if that counts. 'Well that's important to know', says Tim, 'but mostly I mean treatments for your back'.

And with that, he invites you to lie down and you have your first Bowen treatment. As Tim said, you didn't feel much at all, and felt quite glad that he'd told you, otherwise you would have been disappointed. After a while Tim says he's finished and begins making notes while you get off the couch and put on your shoes.

'How was that?' asks Tim. 'Fine' you say 'but I didn't feel anything'. 'That's ok, that's usual' Tim reassures you. 'However, over the next few days you might notice all sorts of strange things. I didn't want you to be alarmed, but if you could make a note of them, to remember to tell me next time? 'Like what?' you ask, worried. 'Oh, like you might feel a bit more sleepy or thirsty for a day or two. Some people feel a bit achy or slightly under the weather for 24 hours. Or you might not feel any of those things. Most people do feel a marked improvement in their symptoms, though. There isn't a right or wrong way, only the way your body chooses to heal'. And with that, he gets his appointment diary to make another date, you pay him and leave.

Second Scenario

You arrive at the clinic a bit early, not wanting to be late for your 10 o'clock appointment. The receptionist spends so long trying to find your name in the appointment book that you wonder if you've got the wrong day. She asks you to take a seat. 10 o'clock comes and goes. At twenty past, you go over and ask if you've got the wrong time. 'Oh' she says 'Tim must be running late, as usual.' Feeling a bit cross, as well as apprehensive about this unknown treatment, you sit back and wait.

At 10:30, Tim comes in looking harassed, throws you a glance, says 'Hi, Come on' and just about waits for you to follow him. When you walk into the treatment room, he's sitting at the table, pen in hand, ready to start writing. You sit on the only other chair and he begins to fire questions. 'Name? Date of birth? Address? Your doctor's address? And what's the problem?' You answer him, but the next question comes almost before you've finished speaking. Tim hardly looks at you. He wants to know about the medical tests you've had, asks a couple of questions about your general health and then says 'Right, shoes and jacket off, and lie down on here', gesturing to the treatment couch.

You do as he says, you can feel him touching your back, and then hear him walk out of the room. A bit surprised, you wonder what to do. Has he finished and should you get up? You decide to wait. Tim comes in again, does something else to your back and leaves. Now you're totally bewildered, but remember what your friend's friend said about it working.

Eventually Tim tells you to get up and put on your shoes. He's busy writing. 'You'll need to come see me at least four more times. You mustn't have any other treatment, massage, homeopathy, anything like that at all. Make the appointments with the receptionist. That'll be £30 please'.

The two scenarios are obvious examples of good practice and bad practice, and your own first experience probably fell somewhere in between. You may have been a practice client for a friend who was training. Or you may never have had any Bowen technique until you started training yourself. And I imagine that, if you are a Bowen practitioner, that your own communication style, and the amount of information you give clients, also falls somewhere between the two. But, which of the hypothetical Tim's do you think keeps clients coming back until he has fixed them, and which do you think has a high drop-out rate?

Chapter 18

The Importance of the Client – Practitioner Relationship

Why do increasing numbers of people turn to complementary therapies to ease their suffering? A recent UK government study showed that as many as one in four people now try Complementary and Alternative Medicine (CAM) at some point in their lives. Here are a few reasons why:

1. Some therapies certainly offer things that conventional medicine does not - massage and aromatherapy, for example, may provide a deep sense of relaxation that is not available on the NHS.

2. Some therapies offer pain relief for chronic conditions, which some people prefer to use instead of medication; acupuncture and Bowen Technique are examples.

3. Conventional medicine has limited success treating back pain, one of the major causes of employment sickness, but osteopathy and Bowen Technique are well known for treating the causes.

4. Many are balancing therapies, working with the whole body to induce a sense of well-being and possibly prevent illness, if used regularly. In China, in the old days, people paid their regular acupuncturist to keep them well and stopped when they got sick, thus encouraging the acupuncturist to make them better as soon as possible!

5. Some therapies are based on completely different models of sickness and health and may be seen as an attractive alternative for someone for whom conventional avenues of treatment have been explored without success.

The possibility of a more attentive relationship with a health professional is also a reason people go to a CAM practitioner. With increasing pressure on goals, cost effectiveness and time management, the average practitioner within primary care or at medical specialist level has little time to spend in a consultation to attend to much other than symptom, diagnosis and a treatment decision. In specialist hospital clinics, staffed by junior doctors doing their stint in obstetrics, neurology or rheumatology, the high turnover means that a long term patient may be seen by a different person on each visit.

For years I attended a clinic at a well-known eye hospital for a regular yearly check-up, and I never saw the same clinician twice. Although I was always treated with courtesy and consideration, I had no sense of an ongoing relationship, that the person looking into my eyes knew me or my personal and medical history.

In a way we've all got used to the 'doctor as technician' model. The image of the paternal general practitioner who was doctor to the same community for most of his working life (I'm using the male deliberately here, because at that time the doctor was much more likely to be a man), who knew the children in each family because he may even have delivered them, who was known, reliable and trusted, is the stuff of myth and old time movies.

My grandfather was one of these old timers; he'd been in practice in East London for thirty years, along with two brothers. In his early days, long before the advent of the National Health Service, he kept his own pharmacy that consisted (or so the story goes) of green pills and blue pills, both of which were placebos. The real healing came from my grandfather's presence and his ability to listen and remember. He had a relationship with each and every one of his patients. He also performed minor surgery, could identify the moment when a person sick with pneumonia would recover or die, and knew the importance of carbolic soap.

There's a way in which we have all got used to the ten minute appointment with the doctor during which the computer screen vies with us for the doctor's attention. And maybe this doesn't matter if the problem is a skin rash, or we need a sick note, or a referral to a specialist. But imagine you'd just got pregnant and weren't sure you wanted to keep the baby, or were worried that the lump on you breast was cancer, or that you're going mad. Wouldn't you want a different kind of attention? Someone who looked and listened, not just to the symptoms, but also to information about you, in order to ascertain what support structure you had, how you were coping and what else they could do for you? The thing that CAM practitioners can still afford to offer, many of us working in private practice with patients who can afford to pay for our time as well as our skills, is the twenty first century equivalent of the old 'bedside manner'.

There's evidence to show that this kind of attentive relationship is one of the things that attracts people to complementary therapies. And in the psychotherapy and counselling world with its burgeoning number of different schools, models and theories, research has shown, time and again, that the most important factors in a successful outcome are the willingness of the client to participate and the nature of the relationship between client and therapist. The actual model used seems to make little difference.

The recent exception to this is the HPC (Health Professions Council) study that found that CBT (Cognitive Behavioural Therapy) far exceeded other psychological therapies for success rates. There are several good reasons for this finding, which include the fact that CBT is, as the name suggests, a behavioural therapy involving the establishment of a clear objective treatment goal for the client. It is far easier to measure, say, ability to travel three steps on the underground in a person with acute travel phobia, than to measure success in a client with repeated abandonment issues from childhood and a history of depression, who finds intimate relationship difficult. Or someone who is facing death from a terminal illness, or an asylum seeker who is not only living with an unfamiliar culture, but has witnessed his family murdered.

CBT does have a high success rate, but another element to take into account is that practitioners can be selective about who they choose to treat. The client must be motivated and willing to do the homework required alongside the sessions. Clients who aren't prepared to participate fully may not be accepted. So CBT is a highly successful therapy, but with a selected client group, and with specific issues.

But if it is true that the quality of the inter-personal connection between client and practitioner is an important factor in the healing process, then surely it makes sense for CAM practitioners to attend to such matters. No matter what therapy we offer, we are not merely skillful technicians, but the general public turn to us with an expectation that we offer more than a conveyor belt approach to treating their ailments.

I work as a complementary therapist, using massage and craniosacral therapy and as a psychotherapist. Some of my clients just want attention for stiff shoulders while others want me to sit with them while they talk about their lives and difficulties. Some clients lie down and I touch them, others sit opposite me and we never touch. Working in these different fields for over twenty years, I've come to realize that no matter what therapy I'm doing, the one factor that is constant is me and the sort of relationship I have with my clients. And that it matters. Psychotherapists and counselors have always recognized the centrality of the relationship in 'the talking cure', as Freud called it. Many CAM practitioners don't, despite the fact that we may claim to be holistic and take account, when we work, of all aspects of our clients' being.

We all have many sorts of relationships with people. Consider how differently you might act and feel with your mother, a neighbour, an old tutor, your dentist and a baby. Even though you're the same person, there are subtle differences in how you are in the different roles life offers. The therapeutic relationship is one where one person is skilled and qualified to offer assistance of some kind to another person who is suffering or in need of help.

There's a power imbalance in such a relationship, however uncomfortable we may feel with the fact. The person called therapist or practitioner or healer is responsible for deciding what's in the other's - client, patient – best interest, for working ethically, watching the boundaries of the relationship, holding the space, showing respect by listening with care, communicating clearly and dealing with all fairly. The person called therapist has a responsibility for his or her self-care, maintaining a healthy lifestyle so that he or she is fit to work. A practitioner with a bad hangover is not functioning at his optimal best. The person called therapist is also responsible for his or her own thoughts and feelings about clients.

We're human beings; there are bound to be some people who rub us up the wrong way, push our buttons, who we dread seeing in the appointment book. If we just squash our negative feelings, there's a danger that they might just pop out in the session from underneath the calm professional facade. If the person called therapist has some understanding of himself and his inner world there is far less danger of his own feelings interfering in the therapeutic relationship.

I use the person called therapist deliberately to remind us that our position on that side of the fence, as it were, is not fixed. It's important to remember what it feels like to be a client, how hard it can be, at times, to seek or accept help and support, to feel vulnerable. It reminds us to stay sensitive to the predicament of the new client, new to our therapy, to CAM therapies in general, perhaps, and certainly to us as practitioner.

Many of us became complementary therapists because we wanted to help others: helping others makes us feel good. It also makes us feel powerful. There's a fine line between acknowledging this with humility and needing our (sick) clients to make ourselves feel better.

Different levels of the therapeutic relationship

Like the layers of an onion, there are various aspects to the relationship we have with clients. This model of the different levels of the therapeutic relationship is adapted from Petrushka Clarkson's book *The Therapeutic relationship*.

1. The working alliance

This refers to the understanding that is reached during the initial consultation about what is needed and how it's going to be achieved. In a good working alliance, both parties have a degree of confidence and trust in each other. There may be feelings of goodwill, or liking, or respect.

2. The real relationship

This refers to the human relationship, when the practitioner puts aside his professional mask and allows some of his personal self into the relationship. This is a tricky one to manage because sharing personal experience can be helpful, for example if used to normalise a client's concerns, or can be relationship building, or help a shy person relax, but too much can be intrusive or unwanted. I once had an osteopath who spent much of my session talking about her children. I didn't like it at all.

3. The transference – counter-transference relationship

Freud was the first to suggest that unconscious processes are at work in any relationship and this idea has since been elaborated and refined by numerous others. At its simplest, this means that one person transfers his experience of a person from his past (usually a significant adult like a parent) onto another person in the present. This may be partly conscious, but is much stronger than just being reminded of someone, because they share the same hairstyle, for example. It's as if the here and now person, the recipient of the transference, becomes the past person in the mind of the other and he starts to behave and think as he used to with the past person. And the person who receives the transference may begin to feel and act in certain ways towards the other in reaction; this is called the counter transference.

It sounds complicated, but here's an example: James is a tall grey haired chiropractor in his 60's, who wears steel rimmed glasses and waistcoats. He's genuinely interested in his clients and gets many word of mouth referrals. Sonia comes to see him. Although she'd heard good things about him and he seems nice enough, she feels very uncomfortable in his presence and can't relax during the treatment. James finds himself, to his surprise, worrying that he's going to hurt her in some way. Sonia doesn't go for any more treatment. Much later she realizes that James reminded her of an uncle who'd abused her when she was three years old. Because this was unconscious, both parties were affected by the transference, without understanding why.

4. The reparative relationship

As the name suggests, this means the sort of relationship that provides a healing alternative to a former, wounding, one. There are many ways in which the complementary therapy relationship can be reparative: a listening empathic practitioner, who uses touch respectfully, may compensate for painful medical treatment, for example. People who've been traumatized at the hands of others can begin to regain trust that contact won't be hurtful within a complementary therapy relationship.

5. The transpersonal relationship

The transpersonal refers to the spiritual, mysterious, religious - to the times which have a different quality from ordinary day to day experience, which some describe as altered states of consciousness. Both practitioner and client may have strong spiritual beliefs but this doesn't mean that the transpersonal will occur in their working relationship, and, on the other hand, two agnostics may find themselves sharing an out of the ordinary moment.

Chapter 19

Self-care and resources

As CAM practitioners we are concerned with the health and well being of our clients and may give advice about diet, exercise, supplements, meditation and so on, depending on our therapy. How often do you find yourself telling someone to do something and thinking that your advice also applies to yourself? We do have a responsibility, not just to ourselves but also to our clients, to stay healthy and fit to work. I know this is stating the obvious but glance through the following checklist and see how well you do. Be honest!

Basic self-care

1. A good practitioner eats a balanced diet (balanced depends on lifestyle, cultural or religious requirements, age, and belief system – I'm not prescribing!)

2. Does not have eating problems

3. Drinks enough water

4. Uses alcohol in moderation

5. Gets enough sleep

6. Exercises regularly

7. Gets fresh air regularly

8. Knows how to relax and does so, regularly

As well as the obvious, there are ways in which we need to look after ourselves that are specific to our therapy. A chef needs to keep his counters clean and his knives sharp. For complementary therapists, the tools used are their own body and mind. If you practice Bowen all day long you are on your feet much of the time: are your shoes comfortable and sufficiently supportive? Do you use your body ergonomically? Is your couch the right height? How do you stretch between clients to relieve tension from the positions you use to work?

Bowen requires a level of stillness and focus as you palpate and work with the tissues. How do you exercise your mind in order to switch into this level of awareness with ease? Do you have a meditation practice of some kind, or other ways of allowing the monkey mind that chatters away most of the time to shut down?

Resources

And what do you do to help yourself feel good? What makes your heart sing or, at the least, provides respite from the drudgery of day-to-day life? We need to be able to look after ourselves properly for two reasons. Firstly, it's hard not to be affected by the suffering of the people who walk into our treatment rooms and we don't do anyone any favors if we take it on and, worse, take it home at the end of the day. Secondly, a work life that requires giving constantly to others can result in the practitioner feeling depleted, and if the lack isn't made good, resentful. If we have ways of making ourselves feel good, rested, happy, that restores our faith in humanity and the inherent goodness of the world, and if we use them, we aren't being selfish but responsible. And indirectly, it's good for our clients too.

A resource is anything that makes you feel good. It can help to identify them and use them with awareness. For example, for many people a soak in a hot bath is relaxing and pleasurable. One person runs the bath out of habit, gets in and worries abut the day's events. Another takes time to switch off the phone, add scented oils, light a candle and appreciates the feel of warm water easing her tension. Who is going to be more resourced afterwards?

Reflect for a moment and make a list of your own resources. These headings might help:

Objects (like the painting on your kitchen wall)
People (the friend who makes you laugh, no matter how dull you feel)
Activities (sports, gardening, collecting)
Places (being in nature is a resource for many people)
Other things (your cat)

Now go through your list and make a note of how many times you used each one in the last week. Or month? Is there any way you could make more use of your resources?

Professional Resources

As well as keeping ourselves resourced as human beings, we also need to keep our work resourced, to keep ourselves fresh, learning and interested and avoid burn out. There's a saying in the teaching profession that there are teachers who teach for twenty years and those who teach the first year twenty times. Of course we all now have to show evidence of continuing professional development, and this obligation makes it less likely that any of us will be doing the same treatments in twenty years time that we do now.

List your professional resources, using the following headings:

Supervision / mentoring
Getting your own treatments
Reading books or journals
Attending courses
Attending conferences
Discussing work with colleagues

Then go through again and note how many you've used in the past week. Or month? Is there anything you'd like to change?

Ten Reasons why Supervision or Mentoring is a Good Thing

Supervision, mentoring or coaching, all variations of the same activity, are now commonplace in many businesses and organizations and mandatory in many of the helping professions, but not yet in the Bowen world. We've been slow to acknowledge ourselves as fully paid up members of the complementary therapy field, reluctant to own our power and our place as professionals alongside the rest of them. People who help others in a professional capacity need support and help themselves.

The good practitioner accepts that CPD is important to update skills and keep her Bowen practice fresh. I happen to believe that good supervision can also be an invaluable part of any Bowen therapist's work. Here's why:

1. Supervision is supportive, affirming and validating. It isn't the client's job to make us feel good about our work, and many of us work in isolation. Talking to another professional helps, especially when self esteem plummets and we question the value of our work.

2. It provides a reflective space to explore the thoughts and feelings that inevitably arise for anyone in a helping/ caring profession in relation to the people who are being 'helped'. There's a danger that overlooking this material, thinking that it doesn't matter, may result in unintentional spillage into the relationship with the client.

3. It's a forum to discuss the 'difficult' client, which usually means the client that we personally find difficult, and to explore what he or she might be triggering for us, as well as strategies for managing the situation.

4. Many practitioners are sensitive and pick up energies, emotions or somatic sensations from clients. Touching someone usually exaggerates this ability. This can be a gift to the treatment, but a drain on the practitioner who doesn't fully understand what's happening or how to protect herself. Supervision can help with this.

5. Certain client groups – people with cancer, babies, people with sensory deficit, for example - need specialist approaches. Supervision can be a place to discuss these issues and learn new skills.

6. In order to help other people effectively, the therapist has to stay fresh and know how to resource herself. A good supervisor notices when you are becoming tired or jaded with the work.

7. Good supervision helps us work trans-culturally. It allows the space to air openly thoughts or feelings about clients who may be different to us, so that these thoughts

and feelings don't contaminate the working relationship; the body picks up what we feel about it, even if we say nothing.

8. Supervision is a form of personal and professional development. It isn't therapy, but it is a good way to develop self-awareness and the ability to evaluate our strengths and weakness as a practitioner.

9. It can help clarify the sort of muddles that can occur for the practitioner who works within an organization, such as lines of responsibility, communication channels and client confidentiality.

10. Good supervision helps us to work ethically, to adhere to our own values and those of our professional organization, and to avoid the spectre of litigation.

How to find a supervisor

You'll notice that most of the reasons I've given for the benefits of supervision don't actually specify anything about Bowen. I happen to believe that, if someone has had good basic Bowen training, receives treatment regularly for herself and keeps up to date with CPD, supervision isn't necessary as an arena to explore practical skills.

So a supervisor doesn't have to be a Bowen practitioner, although an understanding of the therapy obviously helps. It's relationship matters that supervision can help with; the relationship between practitioner and client, practitioner and organisation, clinic, health centre or other place of work, and the relationship between the practitioner and her own physical, mental and energetic well being. Counsellors and psychotherapists, particularly body psychotherapists, know all about this, and some also have specific training in supervision.

Chapter 20

The Practical Aspects of the Client-Practitioner Relationship

Relationships need attention, we all know that. Take a relationship for granted – forget to send birthday cards, assume that your nearest and dearest will forgive anything, don't phone until you want something –this sort of behaviour leads to resentment and cross words, or the gradual fading out of the connection. The same holds for the therapeutic relationship. Within the psychotherapy world, reams have been written about this particular relationship. Some schools of therapy, the psychoanalytic ones, work almost exclusively with the therapeutic relationship. That is to say, the understanding is that the healing takes place by examining the nature of the way that the patient relates to the analyst in the here and now and analysing such behaviour with reference to events in the past.

Every move that the Bowen practitioner makes is informed by knowledge of the anatomy, particularly of the muscular system and fascia. While learning the technique, some of this knowledge is foreground. The student practitioner is conscious of all the necessary parameters in order to absorb them. But for the experienced practitioner the anatomy and physiology is often background, out of conscious awareness, but there, in the frame, all the same.

Of course, it is conceivable that the Bowen moves could be learned by copying a teacher, with no reference to the underlying structures and without understanding what it is that's being moved. It would be much more difficult to develop a sensitivity to the different layers of tissue. So it is with the more subtle aspects of the client – practitioner relationship. Some understanding of the unconscious aspects of the relationship can inform, add a new dimension and ease the dynamic between practitioner and client and is particularly useful when things go wrong. But there are also the behaviours that we engage in consciously, maybe automatically, as part of how we relate to clients.

Boundaries and Containment

What comes to mind when I mention boundaries? A demarcation line, like the one at the edge of a cricket pitch, which determines whether the batsman gets four or six runs?

Something on an ordinance survey map? A set of rules and regulations? Essentially, a boundary is something that may or may not have a physical reality, but that demarcates one area from another. A cell wall, for example, is the boundary line between the cell contents, cytoplasm, nucleus, endoplasmic reticulum and the intercellular fluid that surrounds it. Most of the contents are contained within the wall, unless it is damaged, but some, like oxygen and carbon dioxide, can move in and out, because the cell wall is also permeable.

Driving through Europe you'll cross the boundaries that separate one country from another; sometimes there might be a physical reality to the boundary, like a river, but more often the line is artificial, made by humans, moveable and invisible. Everyday relationships are governed by the norms that dictate the sort of behaviours that are acceptable within the boundary and those that are 'out of line'.

When I think about boundaries as they apply to my work as a complementary therapist I think first of literal, physical boundaries, the 'cell wall' of my work, and then of the relationship boundaries. My 'cell wall' consists of the building of the practice where I work and, inside that, my treatment room. Both are permeable – people come in and out – but it's essential, I think, for the safety and wellbeing of my clients that the boundary to my treatment room is not permeable while I'm working. I don't want anyone else to come in, so I put a large 'engaged' sign on the door.

I once did a little informal research amongst my colleagues, asking them if they'd ever experienced a time with a complementary therapist that they felt showed lack of awareness of professional boundaries. Several people described situations where other practitioners or receptionists had come in and out of the room during their session with a therapist. Most said that the disruption made them feel very unsafe.

Not only does a session with a client take place within a prescribed physical boundary, it also occurs within a set time limit. The time given for the beginning of the appointment and the time it finishes are also boundaries. Clients are always given an appointment time, but how often do we remember to give first time clients the end time as well? And does it matter? If we believe, as the poet Robert Frost pointed out, that 'good boundaries make good neighbours,' that secure boundaries are an important part of any professional relationship, then it makes sense that the client knows when he or she will be leaving. Some of the items in the lists below – contracting and client records - include legal requirements as well as being good professional practice.

Good Boundary Checklist

Your treatment room

1. Is it quiet – not disturbed by the sound of other practitioners working, or music, or loud traffic?

2. Is it comfortably warm?

3. Is it well ventilated?

4. Is the door secure when you're with a client so that no one else can come in?

5. Is your mobile phone or landline turned off or set to silent?

Time

1. Do you begin sessions at the appointed time?

2. Do you let clients know how long a session lasts?

3. Do you end on time, or at least inform your client if you have to run over time?

4. If a client is having a series of treatments, are you able to offer the same time on the same day?

Money

1. How do you inform your clients about your charges? In writing, on leaflets or a website? Verbally, at the time of making an appointment? Via a receptionist? At the end of the session?

2. What do you do about cancellations? Are clients informed about payment for cancellations when they book?

3. What do you do about non-payment?

Contracting

1. Do you explain to the client what the Bowen technique is and what it can do?

2. Do you tell them about other therapies that could also treat the same condition?

3. If you offer more than one therapy yourself, how do you communicate this to a client?

4. How do you know that a client has understood and accepted the treatment you are offering, and the terms of the treatment (cost, number of sessions)?

Client Records

1. Do you keep all identifiable information about a client – name, address, contact details, GP, date of birth – separate from case notes?

2. Do you keep notes on each session?

3. Do you keep client notes in a secure place that no unauthorised person can access?

4. Do you keep client notes for the recommended number of years after termination of treatment? (usually seven – check with your insurer or professional body)?

5.   Are you registered with the Data Protection Registrar?

Professional Boundaries

The next level of boundaries to be considered is the behavioural one. We talk about 'behaving professionally' but what does it mean? There's an assumption that once we get the qualification, find a place to practice, start seeing clients, that we'll just know how to behave in relation to our clients. I was certainly never taught how to do this. Like most practitioners, I suppose, I modelled my behaviour on what I observed in my tutors, and the practitioners I went to for treatment. To demonstrate that professional behaviour is different from everyday behaviour, even if subtly, I invite you to imagine the following scenarios:

1.   You've invited friends for a celebration. The doorbell goes, and you answer. What might you say? Notice your facial expression and body language.

2.   You're waiting with other people, sitting on chairs, outside a door waiting for an interview. The door opens, someone comes out and calls your name. You stand up. What do you say? Notice your facial expression and body language.

3.   You're waiting in your treatment room for a new client and there's a knock on the door. Or you go to reception, or whatever the setup is for meeting new clients at the place where you work. Notice your facial expression and body language.

Here's another exercise that might help you clarify what you consider to be professional (or unprofessional) behaviour. Don't think too hard when you read this list; notice your gut reactions.

1.   It's all right for practitioners to shake hands with a new client when they meet them.

2.   It's all right for practitioners to wear shorts and flip-flops to work.

3. It's all right for practitioners to phone clients at home for a chat.

4. Professional behaviour means never telling a client anything about your personal life.

5. It's all right to hug your client.

6. Practitioners should never have sex with clients that they're currently treating.

7. It's all right for practitioners to ask favours of their clients.

8. Practitioners should always wear a white coat.

9. Professional behaviour means not being too friendly with a client in the treatment room.

10. It's all right to meet clients for coffee or a drink.

You probably found your answers ranging between yes, no and maybe. While there are no right answers for most of these – even item six could be permissible if the client in question is your wife – most of them depend on circumstance. For example, it may feel appropriate to hug a long standing client who is finishing treatment because he's moving out of the area, and you'll probably never meet again, but it wouldn't be acceptable to hug every client at the end of a session. People vary in their preferred style as well. Some practitioners are naturally reserved, and prefer a formal manner, while those of a more gregarious nature might be more informal. It is a question of finding the balance, one that suits you, between professional and friendly, while recognising clearly which behaviours are 'out of bounds' for a complementary therapist. If you're not sure, read your code of ethics.

Clear Communication

There's another aspect to the relationship between client and practitioner that is a factor in the professional behaviour, but isn't to do with the boundaries. Communication is about what happens within the boundaries, and it is the job of the practitioner, not the client, to be able to communicate clearly. We tend to think of communication in terms of talking, but it also involves listening to what is being communicated, and understanding it. Which all sounds very obvious, but can, in the treatment room – as in any aspect of our lives, be open to all sorts of misunderstandings. Read the following extract as if it's a reply from a new client to your question 'What's the problem?'

'Well, it all went bad last Thursday, so I thought I should call someone, but my wife said go to the doctor but I wasn't going to listen to her, since the accident she's been even more nervous than usual. By tea time the pain got so awful. At first it was a niggle, but the insurance doctor said see an osteopath, but my mate Alan, he came to you, that was before the accident, you fixed his back. And last Thursday I fell off the ladder and here I am'.

What do you understand to be the problem? This hypothetical client isn't a good communicator. But as practitioner it's your job to understand what he's saying. Listening carefully we notice that:

1. He fell off his ladder last Thursday.

2. His friend came to see you, and you fixed him.

3. There seems to have been an accident prior to the fall from the ladder, but it's not clear.

We can assume from 2 that he's chosen to see you with an expectation that you can fix him too, but we still don't know what the problem is, or the nature of the accident that may have triggered it. So we ask the relevant questions, and listen to the answers, until we have all the information needed to do the treatment.

As well as listening to the words and the content of what our clients communicate, it's important to 'listen' to what might be being communicated non-verbally. If our hypothetical client were speaking very rapidly, leaning forward on the edge of his chair, he'd be communicating nervousness, or anxiety, but if his speech was ponderous, with long pauses, monotone and hard to hear, we might make different assumptions about his mental and emotional health. Either way, we'd adjust our behaviour and way of communication in response to his. At least we would if we were good communicators.

Listening Skills Check List

1. Do you wait until a client has finished speaking before you reply or ask the next question?

2. Do you listen differently to clients than you do to friends?

3. Do you listen to the meaning behind the words as well as their content?

4. Are you able to put your own concerns on one side when you listen to a client?

5. Do you sometimes jump to conclusions and stop listening?

6. Can you respect what your client says even when you don't agree?

Clear Communication Check List

1. Are you able to say what you mean in a few words ?

2. Is your speaking voice loud and clear enough for most people to hear without straining?

3. Do you make appropriate eye contact with clients? (remember that 'appropriate' is dependant on cultural background.)

4. Do you try to match the words you use to the client's level of understanding and experience?

Working with Vulnerable Clients

Here are some pointers to help you adapt how you communicate and / or treat clients who are vulnerable.

Physical Vulnerability

Clients who are 'physically vulnerable' range from the person with a leg in plaster after a sports accident, to the permanently disabled person with cerebral palsy, to the elderly client who can no longer walk unaided. Many of these suggestions also apply to the very elderly, but please remember that old age is NOT a disease state but something that will, in time, happen to you too.

1. Be sensitive to the emotional and psychological aspects of living with a physical impairment.

2. Don't infantilise.

3. Remember that people who have had to endure a lot of medical touch may not have much experience of choosing what happens to their body. It may help to explain more carefully than usual what the treatment entails and why, and that the person can make choices about how she is touched and where.

4. Make an assessment of need before the first attendance. Does the client require wheel chair access, for example?

5. Allow more time for the initial consultation and for dressing and undressing.

6. Be prepared to adapt how you work and negotiate with your client about where would be most comfortable to be treated – in a chair or on the couch – and how to position and support his body.

7. If there is sensory loss he may not be able to give accurate feedback.

8. Ask the client where he would like any equipment
    - braces, breathing apparatus, chair, walking stick - ask

where he would like them to be during the treatment.

9.   If he has incontinence problems, be sensitive to potential embarrassment, and straightforward about discussing practical possibilities.

Dyslexia

1.   If you ask clients to read and fill in medical histories or consent forms remember that a dyslexic client may find this hard.

Communication Difficulty

Communication involves the ability to understand language and the ability to produce meaningful speech. Some clients, people with Down's syndrome for example, may have limited ability in both areas. Someone who has had a stroke may have perfectly good understanding but have slurred speech. A client whose mother tongue is not English may have limited ability to communicate, but this doesn't mean she is stupid.

1.   Be sensitive to confidentiality issues if an advocate, family member or translator accompanies the client to speak for him.

2.   Include the client as much as possible in the consultation, to avoid the 'Does he take sugar?' situation.

3.   Face the client and make use of facial expression and gesture, and use simple language if he has a comprehension difficulty.

4.   If the client's speech is hard to understand, allow time, ask for clarification and repeat what's been said to check if you've got it right. Don't pretend to understand if you don't.

5.   Explain as clearly as you can what will happen.

6.   Allow more time for aftercare as well as the initial consultation.

Visual Impairment

1. Ask if the client would like to remove contact lenses or glasses before treatment. Make sure they are put within reach.

2. For people with a severe impairment, keep the layout of the room the same or tell the client if items have been changed.

3. If someone cannot see what you are doing, or what you want him to do, talk it through clearly. Ask him how much assistance he would like moving around the room and getting on and off the couch.

Hearing Impairment

1. Remember, most elderly people have some degree of hearing loss.

2. Make sure your face is visible so that the person can lip read easily. Keep your face in the light, don't cover your mouth with your hand, and speak clearly.

3. If the person has a 'good' ear, position yourself to speak to that side.

4. If the client wears aids, ask if he wants to remove them during the treatment but remember that he won't then be able to hear your instructions clearly.

Panic Attacks

1. It's probably sensible to include a question about panic attacks in your consultation so that you are alert to the possibility.

2. If a client begins to panic or have an anxiety attack, she is experiencing extreme sympathetic nervous system arousal. Use any tools you have to help your client reduce arousal. Talk calmly, ask the client to focus on her breathing, help her to slow it down, and to notice things in the room.

3. Many aspects of the treatment situation could act as triggers for arousal in someone suffering from post-traumatic stress; including leaving the room during the session, if this is part of the treatment. Be very careful that the client knows this will happen and why, and maybe arrange to knock when you re-enter. Issues of trust and safety are very important and it helps the client if you are very clear about your boundaries, and maintain a professional relationship.

Crying

1. Emotional release often accompanies release in the tissues.

2. For quiet tears with little noticeable change in breathing, let your client know that you've noticed but keep your response light and neutral. You don't have to stop working.

3. Sobbing or evidence of extreme distress might suggest a pause until the client has recovered enough for you to continue.

4. If she curls on her side it is easier to breathe and usually feels safer. Offer tissues. You don't have to do anything. She may want to talk about it and if so, all you have to do is listen.

5. Find out whether the client has professional help or someone to talk to. If appropriate, refer on to a counselling or psychotherapy agency. Bowen work has the ability to evoke powerful old memories that can be quite shocking, even re-traumatising for the client and if the practitioner isn't qualified to deal with these, which most aren't, it's a professional responsibility to be able to refer on to someone who can.

Post Traumatic Stress

The presence of post traumatic stress may not come up at all during an initial consultation, so when a client has an unexpected reaction during treatment, it is all the more alarming. When someone is exposed to a traumatic situation (a train crash, rape, witnessing a violent attack) his or her sympathetic nervous system goes into high arousal. If the effects are not discharged this arousal gets locked into the system, and can result in post-traumatic stress. The symptoms are the same as for everyday stress but persist in the absence of current triggers, causing sleep and appetite disturbance, problems with attention and ongoing anxiety and distress. One of the best books on the subject is *Babette Rothschild's The Body Remembers. The psychophysiology of trauma and trauma treatment.* 2000. W.W. Norton and Co.

Chapter 21

Unconscious Processes in the Therapeutic Relationship

So far we have considered the obvious factors that contribute to good professional relationships. Now it's time to consider other things - the thoughts, feelings and fantasies that lie, usually, just below the surface, and which represent our accumulated baggage from the past - everything we learned about the world and ourselves in our formative years and which we bring with us into the present moment and our interactions with others.

Unless we've been in therapy or spent years in personal growth or have a permanent life coach, somewhere along the way most of us sometimes find other people – clients, colleagues, teachers, family – troublesome. The difficulty may lie with us or with them or somewhere in the tangled web that is relationship. In our personal life we have choices: to confront or discuss the problem with the other person, decide never to see them again, or resolve to let bygones be bygones. When it comes to clients, the responsibility for the difficulty lies with us. We can't say 'I'd like a little more respect from you please / deal with your anger issue before you make another appointment / I suggest you talk to your therapist about your hostility.'

If things go wrong in our relationships with clients, or colleagues, there are some useful ideas from psychotherapy that may help. One of these is a basic understanding of the concepts of somatic transference and projection, and the skills to work with them when they appear – on your own, not with the client. The other thing that helps is thinking about the proverbial elephant in the corner of every practitioner's treatment room, present but ignored. I believe that these elephants, once named and taken care of, loose their power to suddenly stampede and wreck everything. I'm talking about sex and power. And the concept of the therapist's shadow.

Somatic Transference

In everyday language we refer to these ideas when we talk about ' picking things up' from others. Laughter is infectious, we talk about 'feeling for' another and we know how easy it is to get carried away in the emotion of a crowd. Neuroscience is beginning to show us that what psychotherapy calls unconscious process has a somatic component that can actually start in the body. Our nervous, endocrine and muscular systems can mirror those of another person, thereby enabling us to 'know' what he's feeling.

Suppose your client is feeling angry; his facial muscles will tighten or relax into a predictable pattern, as will other muscles in the body, and his autonomic nervous system will trigger predictable changes in heart rate, breathing, tension in his gut muscles and so on. Certain neurochemicals associated with anger will pour into his bloodstream. If he feels happy, a completely different, but also predictable, set of muscular responses and internal changes will occur.

You can try this relationship between external, muscular, and internal for yourself. Right now, contract your risorius muscles – smile! Notice any changes in your gut, chest, breathing pattern. What feeling do you usually associate with these sensations?

The observable muscular patterns of another person can be consciously copied, but it appears that we also copy each other's body movements unconsciously. Scientists have discovered the presence of nerves in the brain that they call mirror neurons. These are motor nerves that fire when watching another person perform a particular action, as if the person watching were doing the action herself. So, if you watch someone break into a big grin and refrain from copying, the neurons that contracted your risorius muscle a moment ago will be firing, as if you were grinning too. So it seems that our bodies copy the body of another person on many different levels and this may be the basis of transference and countertransference, and evidence that we may indeed pick things up from our clients, and them from us.

Here are some examples: A colleague of mine works with anorexic women. At the end of each session she is often starving hungry, even if she knows she has a full stomach. I used to struggle not to fall asleep when sitting with one of my clients until he began to talk about what terrified him – as if his terror was paralysing me, too. If I'm using craniosacral therapy with a client who's recently had anaesthetic, my mind goes foggy and vague. Have you ever had a strange or uncomfortable or powerful reaction to a person and been puzzled by it? Much of the time we can remain puzzled, can manage to get on with the person anyway, or he moves out of our life and no harm's done. But when it comes to clients, or colleagues, this unconscious/somatic transference reactions can get in the way. If we have negative feelings about someone, no matter what the source, the other person can pick it up. Here are some exercises that can help.

Dealing with your own Difficult Feelings

1. Make a list of all the clients / colleagues who you've found difficult. Do it without thinking. At this stage it doesn't matter why.

2. Then next to each name write the reasons why you found that person difficult, something about how they behaved, their attitudes, mannerisms, or how you felt with or after seeing them.

3. Is there a pattern that emerges?

Some people are truly hard to be with, for whatever reason, but often the people we find difficult are those that trigger difficult feelings. They mirror something about ourselves that we don't like or show us a quality that we'd like to have.

The following exercises can be used to make sense of the difficulties. Remember, these tools are for you to use on your own, to be your own supervisor if you like, or a detective looking for clues to solve a mystery. These are not things to discuss with your client. Choose one person from your list.

Talking to your Client as if...

Talking to your client comes from Gestalt therapy and is called 'two-chair work'.

1. You sit opposite an empty chair or cushion and imagine the person you are having difficulties with sitting on the other one. Bring them to mind as clearly as you can.

2. Then imagine what you would like to say to him or her as if he was really there and as if you weren't really a

careful responsible practitioner. You can say anything you like – what you think of the person, how you feel when with them, what it is you can't stand about them, and so on. Continue until you've run out of things to say. This may be sufficient to shift your feelings, but there is a further step you can take.

3.   Change chairs (cushions) and sit in the client's seat. Take a while to settle and be aware of how your body feels in this place, as if you were your client.

4.   Listen to what you can remember from the other side, what you just said and notice your reactions.

Take some time to absorb what happens and then consider the following questions:

1.   How do you feel about your client now? At times, just venting can be enough to shift feelings.

2.   Is there anyone that your client reminds you of? It may be that the strength of your reaction to this person lies in the way she reminds you of someone with whom you have or have had a strong emotional tie. If this is the case, look again at your client on the chair and say very clearly that you know your client is not your father / last head teacher / Mrs Thatcher. If this sounds too easy or a bit silly, it is both – but it can work!

Writing a Letter

If the exercise above sounds impossibly embarrassing or difficult, another way of doing pretty much the same is to write a letter to the client / colleague, saying exactly whatever you like. This is not a letter to send, but one where you can let go of your thoughts and feelings. Don't think too hard about it. Allow your pen to race across the page, or hands to skim over the keyboard without your inner censor getting in the way. Write until you've finished then consider the questions above.

At the end of this exercise, it's good practice to destroy written material or delete it from your computer, just in case anyone should take it for case notes.

Focusing

Focusing is another way to explore what's going on, particularly if you experience the difficulty in a diffuse way that's hard to get a handle on, a sense that things aren't right rather than a clear idea why a person upsets you. It's also a good exercise for those who find it easy to relate to internal sensation.

1. Sit quietly and comfortably and let yourself settle.

2. Bring your 'difficult' client to mind, imagine what he/she looks like, and remember the last session.

3. Now turn your attention inwards, to your own body. What's going on? Scan your body and notice if there's a particular area or sensation that is calling your attention to it.

4. Focus on this sensation and wait. Don't try and think about it or what it means, just be with it. Wait for thoughts or other sensations or emotions to arise.

5. Maintain a patient, interested curiosity with regard to your inner sensations. Allow them to speak to you. Ask them what they mean – be careful not to let your head get in there and decide for them!

Using Images

If you visualise easily, this is a good exercise for you.

1. Sit quietly and comfortably and let yourself settle.

2. Imagine you are sitting in a little film studio, just you and a projector. Or sitting facing your computer screen.

3. Bring your 'difficult' client to mind, imagine what he/she looks like, and remember the last session.

4. Then ask for an image of your client to be shown on the screen.

5. Wait. Just allow whatever emerges. What's your reaction to this image? Do you like it? Does it make any sense to you? Does it help you understand your client or what's going on any better?

If the image isn't particularly helpful, sit with it for a while to see if any insights occur at a later moment.

Sex in the Therapeutic Relationship – How to Work Safely

One person has permission to ask all kinds of intimate information about the other, invites her to lie down, maybe removing some clothes, and touches her body. The other person isn't allowed to do the same. Power imbalance? Of course there is. Some aspects reminiscent of a sexual relationship? Of course. And , of course, no complementary therapist would ever abuse their power or have a sexual relationship with a client, would they? So we don't need to talk about these matters.

Sexual energy and life force energy are powerful forces. They are also natural forces, in the sense that sex is biology and the desire to create life is also a biological imperative, one that all other mammals have no qualms about pursuing, when the urge takes them. Our bodies are designed to have sexual feelings – and thoughts that come with the feelings. And there is nothing wrong with that. How many times have you heard a colleague own up to feeling attraction to a client, or done so yourself? It's sort of taboo, yet if we could talk about these matters there's probably less likelihood that we'd act on them.

Can we acknowledge sexual energy, our own or our clients' and stay within therapeutic boundaries, both professional and personal? Here are some guidelines.

1. Remember, sex is an energy, it is not wrong and it does not have to be acted upon, just experienced. It is also the responsibility of the person experiencing it.

2. A client may have sexual feelings as a response to treatment – a biological response or an energetic release. If this happens and you feel able to accept this, don't shame or blame the client, and if necessary state your boundaries, to remind both of you of the safety of the relationship.

3. If you aren't comfortable with clients' sexual feelings then refer them on. It isn't good practice to work outside your comfort zone. Talk to colleagues, or your supervisor.

4. Sometimes it just isn't clear where the feelings belong. If there is sexual energy around you may be picking it up, or it may be your own biological response. Try these tools to sort out what's going on: refocus your own intention on the work you are doing, on your purpose with the client. If you work with energy, acknowledge the feelings and let them go into the earth. If you normally talk with your client during the treatment, you could try asking what's going on for them, what are they feeling? Sometimes naming something helps disperse it.

5. If you've tried the above and the feelings are still there, or you find yourself thinking sexually about a client outside of sessions, you are not necessarily doing anything wrong. However, research into abuse of clients by psychotherapists suggests that risk factors include having sexual thoughts and feelings about clients, in conjunction with social isolation or going through a period of distress or crisis. If any of this applies, or you find yourself taking more care of your appearance with a certain client, going over time, being lenient about money, talking about yourself more than usual, flirting and not talking about this client in supervision, then you are at risk of inappropriate sexual behavior.

6. What to do? If possible, stop working with the client and get help; talk to a senior colleague or find a supervisor. Remind yourself of your professional responsibilities by reading your professional code of conduct. Try an affirmation such as 'There's nothing

wrong with sexual feelings but I do not have sexual contact with clients.' And finally, find more ways to get your needs for contact and intimacy met in your personal life.

Biography

Su Fox is a Massage, Craniosacral and Psychotherapist in private practice in London and an Assessor for The Massage Training Institute. She is co-author, with Darien Pritchard, of *Anatomy, Physiology and Pathology for the Massage Therapist* and author of *Practical Pathology for Massage*, and *Relating to Clients: the Therapeutic Relationship for Complementary Therapists*, published by Jessica Kingsley. She also offers supervision and can be contacted on *sufox@blueyonder.co.uk*

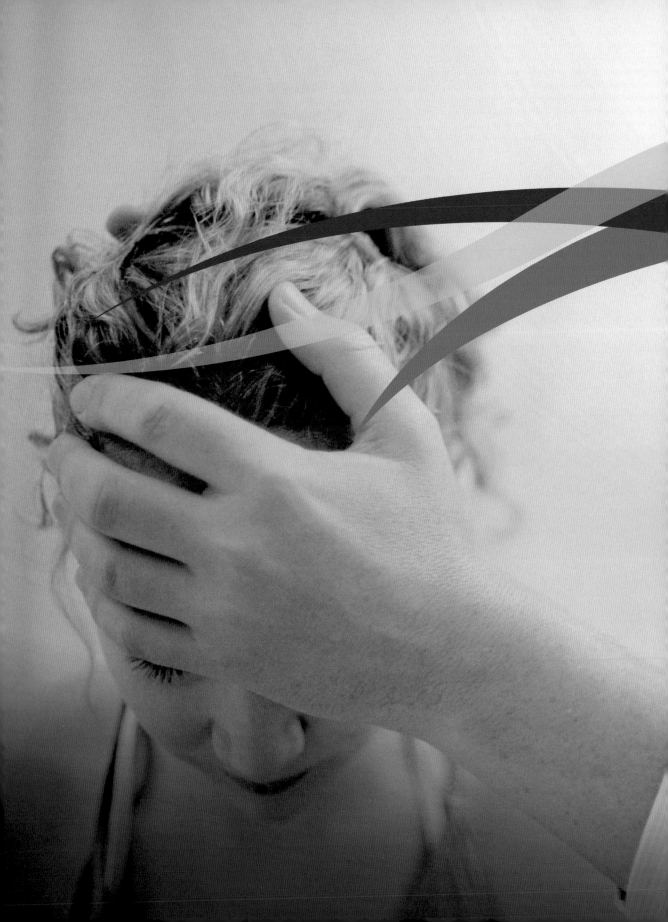

epilogue

Chapter 22

Where do we go from here?

Honouring and trusting not only our own abilities as therapists but also the technique, the innate healing ability of our clients and the higher principles at work, is key to being a good therapist. For some of us, perhaps, the balance can be a little off kilter. We all know therapists who have a little too much belief in their own abilities and perhaps less faith in the technique, or others who don't have enough trust in their clients' innate ability to heal and so work them too hard. Getting the balance right between how much to do, how much to trust, and when to intervene is a lifetime's work.

"Your intelligence is always with you, overseeing your body, even though you may not be aware of its work.... Your intelligence is marvellously intimate. It's not in front of you or behind, or to the left or the right." – *Jelaluddin Rumi, translated by Coleman Barks*

One of the questions I constantly ask myself when treating a client is – 'How can I get this person's body to accept the work?' For some clients a firmer pressure is more suitable because that is what they are comfortable with. A man who is used to a firm massage might feel threatened by a touch that he feels is too 'effeminate'. For others, the lightest of touch will feel too invasive. The question is when you are applying pressure to a muscle - does it resist you? – can it let you in?

The phrase that comes to my mind when I treat clients is one of Dr Sutherland's, the founder of cranial osteopathy. He used to describe his hands as 'all seeing, all sensing, all feeling'. Another image I like is to feel my hands like the paws of a big cuddly teddy bear – teddy bears have big hearts, their paws are warm and soft and they don't have any bones!

"Know your anatomy and your physiology, but when you get your hands on a patient's body, never forget that a living soul dwells therein." – *Dr Andrew Taylor Still, founder of osteopathy*

Can we Listen more?

"There is no greater healing than being heard. The greater
the depth of the hearing, the greater the healing. If I can be
sufficiently present in myself at a deep enough level I can hear
another at a level at which there is only health. We have only to
give up doing anything, we have only to learn to be. Not to be
perfect, just to be." – *Mike Boxhall RCST*

Our ability to 'hear' our clients is predominantly limited by our
belief system and, to a much lesser extent, our skill. In turn, skill
is dependent on how much we use our more subtle faculties and
trust our ability to 'tune in and listen'. By 'hearing' and 'listening'
I mean using all our senses, not just our ears. We are listening
to our clients' life story as it is expressed in their body – the way
they hold it, their pain, their vitality, their relationship to who
they think they are, to where they think they are going, to where
they feel they have come from, their ancestral line, their friends,
their ambitions and their beliefs.

Our bodies are highly sensitive, finely tuned machines and we
are much more sensitive to body language than we give ourselves
credit for. A recent study at the University of California in Los
Angeles (UCLA) found that up to 93 percent of communication
is determined by non-verbal cues.

Unfortunately nowadays there is a prevalent cultural mistrust of
anything that cannot be measured with a scientific instrument,
even though we might have a 'gut feeling' about something. This,
mixed with a desire for profit, has led to some strange anomalies
in our healthcare system - for example midwives being told to
advise breast feeding women to use a proprietary brand of cream
for sore nipples rather then vitamin E cream, even though in
their experience the latter works better.

It would appear that healing takes place primarily through a
person being heard and the client / practitioner relationship
makes this uniquely possible. The practitioner is able to observe
dispassionately, objectively and without judgement, so that it is
quite possible that when we treat a client it may be the first time
in their lives that they feel (even if not consciously) truly listened

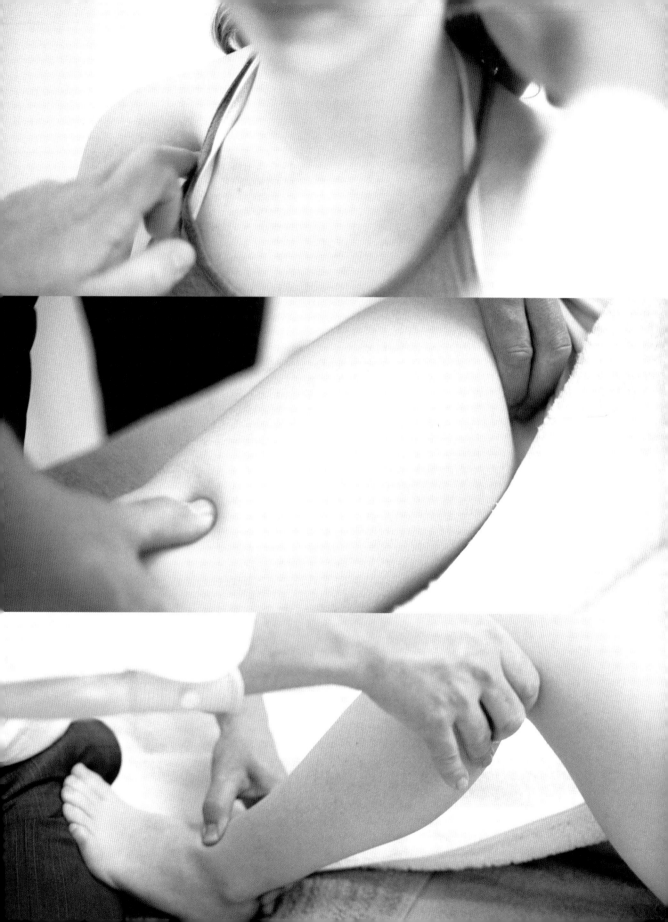

to. In that listening, a letting go and a moving on is made possible on every level, including physically.

"The way in which I relate to others is a most powerful reflection in the most fundamental relationship of all, and that is with myself" – *Tony Parsons, The Open Secret*

Can we be more creative?

Bowen is an incredibly new therapy and the scope for development is huge. In every modality there are strong personalities teaching the work, advocating their approach over another, and Bowen certainly has its fair share of these. Because there are so many apparently conflicting approaches using harder or softer touch, less or even no challenge, longer or non-existing breaks, it would be useful to have some consensus about what works and what doesn't and perhaps some understanding of why.

Some of the most interesting 'advanced' moves have come from the notebooks that Oswald Rentsch kept from his time with Tom Bowen. These include fascinating concepts such as holding a long challenge and moving over the origins and insertions of muscles in opposing directions at the same time, moving directly over nerves and joints, extra moves for the coccyx, the neck, and the TMJ. Constructive discussion amongst those people who are advocating developments to the work, together with a rigorous clinical evaluation of these developments, would be invaluable. Without it, practitioners are likely to become confused and the therapy will factionalise.

If in doubt – pray!

Hopefully this book will have gone some way to making you a better therapist – at least that was the intention! However, reading someone else's ideas is no substitute for the unerring truth that the answer to any question, however difficult, is always available if we are receptive or bother to ask. One of the most beautiful concepts in Cranial Osteopathy is about shifting one's awareness when one is working to see if one can sense another pair of hands working alongside ours. These hands are the real teacher and they are always available.

Of course, as the following illustrates, the key is asking the right question:

Once upon a time, a man was walking through a forest in the Rockies. He was a staunch atheist and had been all his life. As he turned a corner, a large brown bear was blocking his path. The bear looked hungry and began to approach him. The man was understandably terrified and began to run. Unfortunately the bear was faster and began gaining on him rapidly. In desperation the man began to pray - 'God, if you are there, I am truly sorry that I have never believed in you but please find it in your heart to save me from this bear.' A big booming voice came from the sky 'You had many chances to do good deeds in your life but you chose to ignore me. I'm afraid it is time to meet your maker.'

The man was stunned but had the presence of mind to ask again – 'OK, God, I know I have ignored you but please could you at least convert the bear to Christianity – after all the bear has done nothing wrong.'

There was a long silence and then came a brief, booming 'OK.' All of a sudden the bear dropped down on its knees, a pious expression came over its face and it clasped its paws together. As it knelt there, its lips began to move gently. The man peered forward to see what it was saying. He managed to lip read:

'For what we are about to receive, may the Lord...'

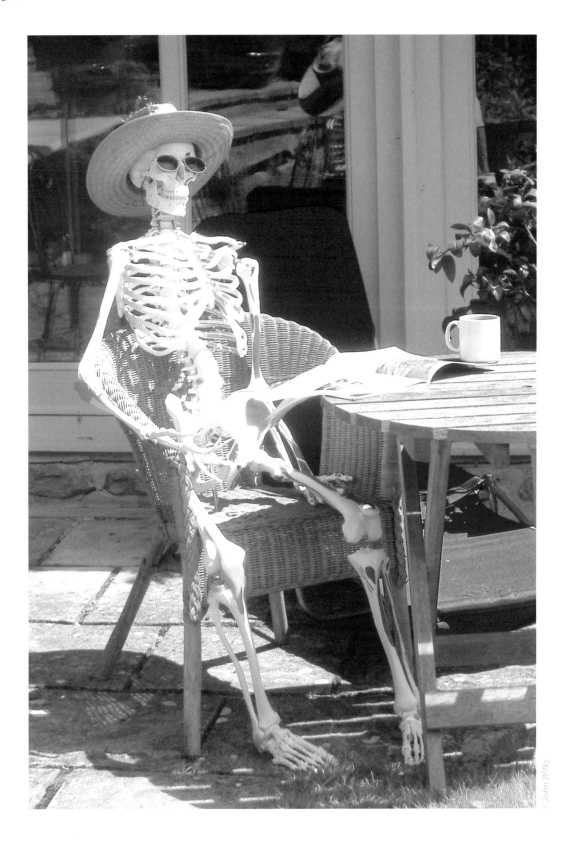

©John Wilks

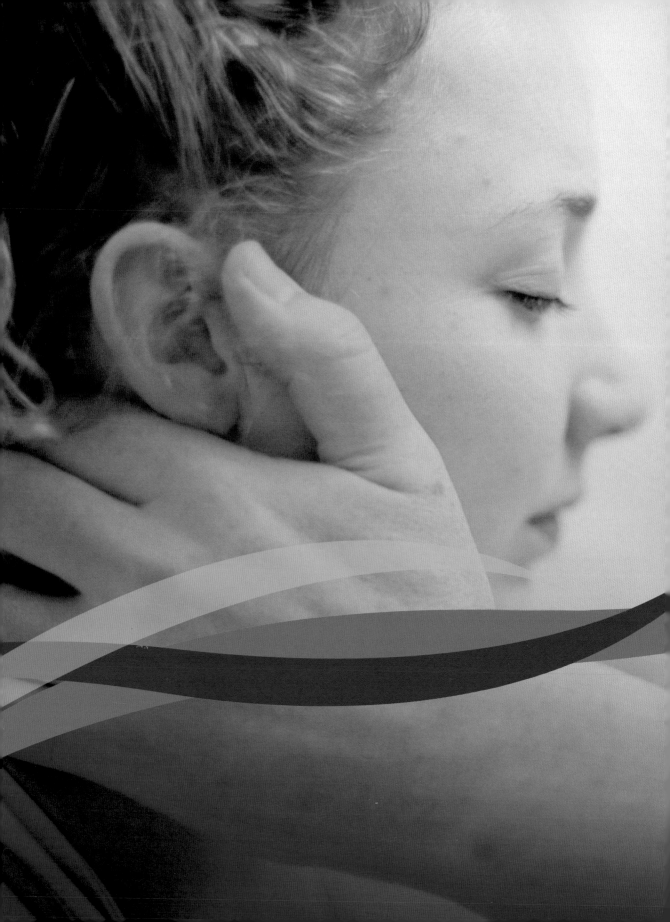

appendices

Appendices

A Note Of Caution

The primary concern of all health professionals is safety, even before efficacy. Knowing when to refer to a doctor, the hospital or another practitioner is a vital skill for any therapist.

In most countries there are certain notifiable diseases where one has a legal obligation to notify the authorities if your client displays classic symptoms of a particular condition. These might include cholera, hepatitis, TB etc. Lists are available from health authorities' websites in each area.

More difficult is the situation where you suspect or are told about physical abuse, particularly in relation to children. Bedwetting, which we see occasionally as Bowen practitioners could, for example, be a sign that a child is suffering abuse. This is more likely in cases of what is termed 'Secondary Bedwetting', which comes on suddenly (and sometimes after an emotional upset like having to go to hospital for an operation, moving schools or some family upset), rather than 'Primary Bedwetting' which can be more simply a developmental issue. In these cases it is essential that you take appropriate action but it is also very important to get legal advice as to the best way to proceed because it is a potential minefield for all concerned.

In other situations one might notice a suspected melanoma – for example you might be working on someone who lives alone and notice an irregular shaped blemish on the skin.

Balancing the need for the person to seek medical help without alarming them is always difficult but it is essential that the person wastes no time in getting help as melanomas can spread to the deeper tissues very quickly and then be much more difficult to treat. As a practitioner it is worth familiarising yourself with what melanomas look like and their characteristics.

Cancers and tumours are notoriously difficult to diagnose sometimes, and in any case it is not our job to diagnose. There is a variety of different areas that people might get tumours – for example prostate or ovarian cancer will often spread to the pelvic bowl; tumours on the spine, the ilia or even the spinal cord itself are possible. However, there are certain tell-tale signs that might give you cause for concern and you will need to ask the person to get a second opinion.

Possible symptoms someone might exhibit may include any or all of the following:

- The person responds slightly to treatment but not significantly or the symptoms keep coming back

- The pain is unrelenting, even if not particularly bad, and is not so dependent on what activity they do. It might be worse at night

- They may have changes in other ways – a loss of weight, change in digestion (constipation or diarrhoea), abdominal bloating, bladder or bowel discomfort or other unusual symptoms

- Sciatic pain down both legs and/or saddle anaesthesia

Other situations where Bowen may not be so effective are where there is an exitosis (bony outgrowth) on one of the vertebrae which is pressing on one of the nerve roots. The person will usually experience continual pain, and may even suffer from muscle wastage in one leg. Although some Bowen practitioners do have success with this, as it is essentially due to undue strain being put on certain areas of the vertebrae due to postural problems, surgery is sometimes inevitable.

The above list is not exhaustive, so if in doubt always refer on to someone who is qualified and ideally sympathetic to holistic ways of working. The same is true as a general rule for anything for which you are not qualified, such as dietary or exercise advice. Knowing a good naturopath, homeopath, Pilates or yoga teacher near you to whom you can refer clients and who understands the way you work is invaluable.

Please note that this book is not designed to offer advice on your health or that of your clients and that one should always seek the advice of a medically qualified practitioner.

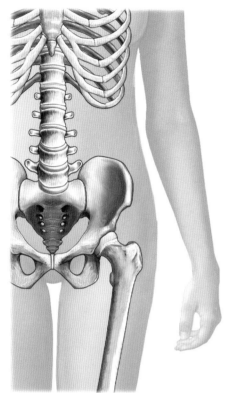

Normal bone matrix

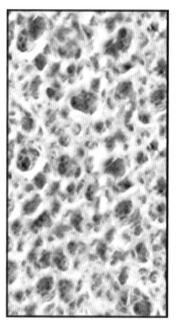

Osteoporosis

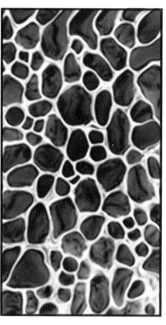

Contact Details

Head Office in Australia

The Bowen Therapy Academy of Australia
P.O. Box 733, Hamilton, Vic. 3300 AUSTRALIA

Phone: (03) 55 723000
From outside Australia dial +61 3 5572 3000

Email: bowtech@h140.aone.net.au
Web: www.bowtech.com

UK Office

The Bowen Association UK and Bowen Training UK
PO Box 4358
Dorchester
Dorset
DT1 3FD, UK

Tel 0700 BOWTECH (0700 269 8324)
From outside the UK dial +44 1305 268936

Email: office@bowen-technique.co.uk
Web: www.bowen-technique.co.uk and
www.bowentraining.co.uk

John Wilks MA RCST BTAA
Wyndham Barns
Corton Denham
Sherborne
Dorset
DT9 4LS

Tel: 01963 220991
Mobile: +44 7866 764 960

Email: mail@jwilks.co.uk
Web: www.therapy-training.com

Ordering

The Bowen Technique – The Inside Story by John Wilks

Cost £25.00 plus p & p of £3.50 per book (1st class post) = £28.50 made payable to **CYMA Ltd**. Please enquire for postage costs overseas, local distributors and bulk orders.

Go to www.cyma.org.uk and follow links for book orders or contact:

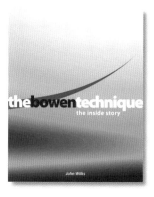

CYMA Ltd
Wyndham Barns
Corton Denham
Sherborne
Dorset
DT9 4LS

Tel +44 (0)1963 220991

Understanding The Bowen Technique and Understanding Craniosacral Therapy by John Wilks

Individual copies from John Wilks at £1.99 each plus p & p of £1.01 per book (1st class post) = £3.00 made payable to **CYMA Ltd**.

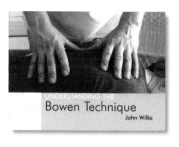 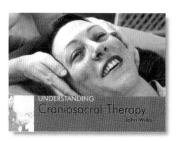

Postage and packing free if ordered with The Bowen Technique - The Inside Story.

ISBN numbers:

Understanding The Bowen Technique	1-904439-36-5
Understanding Craniosacral Therapy	1-904439-35-7
The Bowen Technique – The Inside Story	978-0-9557063-0-1

Bibliography

General Anatomy & Physiology

Essentials of Anatomy & Physiology, Martini F & Bartholomew E, Prentice Hall, 1999

The Principles of Anatomy and Physiology, Tortora G, John Wiley & Sons inc., 1993

Anatomy Atlases

Anatomy, a Regional Atlas of the Human Body, Clemente Carmine D, Urban & Schwarzenberg, 1987

McMinn's Color Atlas of Human Anatomy, Abrahams PH, Hutchings RT, Marks SC, Mosby, 2002

Surface Anatomy- The Anatomical Basis of Clinical Examination (2nd Edition), Lumley J, Churchill Livingstone, 1996

Muscles, Fascia and Connective Tissue

The Muscle Book, Blakey P, Bibliotek Books, 1992

Anatomy Trains, Myofascial Meridians for Manual and Movement Therapists, Myers TW, Elesvier Health Sciences, 2001

The Psoas Book, Koch L, Guinea Pig Productions, 1997

The Trail Guide to the Human Body (Book and DVD), Andrew Biel

Job's Body – A Handbook for Bodywork, Juhan D, Station Hill, 1991

Energy Medicine: The Scientific Basis, Oschman JL, Elsevier Health Sciences, 2000

Assessment

Orthopedic Physical Assessment, Magee DJ, W B Saunders

Exercise

The Egoscue Method of Health Through Motion: Revolutionary Program That Lets You Rediscover the Body's Power to Rejuvenate It (Paperback), Egoscue P, Harper Collins Publishers, 1993

The Autonomic Nervous System

Autonomic Nerves: Basic Science, Clinical Aspects, and Case Studies, Wilson-Pauwels L, B C Decker Inc., 1997

Understanding Trauma

Waking the Tiger – Healing Trauma, Levine P, North Atlantic Books,1997

Mapping the Mind, Carter R, Weideneld & Nicolson, London, 1998

The Emotional Brain, LeDoux J, Phoenix

Molecules of Emotion, why you feel the way you do, Pert C, Simon & Schuster Ltd, 1999

The Body Remembers. The Psychophysiology of Trauma and Trauma Treatment, Rothschild B, W.W. Norton & Co., 2000

The Body Remembers Casebook: Unifying Methods and Models in the Treatment of Trauma, Rothschild B, W.W. Norton & Co, 2003

Babies and Birth

The Mind of Your Newborn Child, Chamberlain D, North Atlantic Books, 1998

Why Love Matters: How Affection Shapes a Baby's Brain (Paperback), Gerhardt S, Taylor & Francis (Routledge), 2004

A Teacher's Window onto a Child's Mind, Goddard SA, Fern Ridge Press, Oregon USA, 1996

Reflexes, Learning and Behaviour, Goddard SA, Fern Ridge Press, Oregon USA, 2001

Human Labor & Birth, Oxorn H, McGraw–Hill Education, Europe, 1985

Women's Health

Your Change Your Choice, Dooley M, Hodder Mobius, 2004

Fit for Fertility, Dooley M, Hodder Mobius, 2007

Nutritional Medicine

Prescription for Nutritional Healing: The A to Z Guide to Supplements, Balch & Balch, Avery Publishing Group, 2002

The pH Miracle, Young R & S, Warner Books Inc., 2003

Osteopathy

Life in Motion, the Osteopathic Vision of Rollin Becker, Becker R, Rudra Press, 1997

The Stillness of Life: The Osteopathic Philosophy of Rollin E Becker, Becker R, Stillness Press

Bowen

Understanding The Bowen Technique, John Wilks, First Stone Pub 2004

Die Original Bowtech Methode, Zainzinger M, & Knoll S, Suedwest- Verlang, 2005

The Therapeutic Relationship

The Therapeutic Relationship in Psychoanalysis, Counseling, Psychology and Psychotherapy, Clarkson P, Whurr, 1995

Focusing, Gendlin ET, Bantam, 1978

Practical Pathology for the Massage Therapist, Fox S, Corpus Publishing Ltd., 2004

Su Fox. Relating to Clients. The Therapeutic Relationship for Complementary Therapists, Jessica Kingsley 2007

Psychotherapy - an Erotic Relationship, Mann D, Taylor & Francis (Routledge), 1997

The Therapeutic Relationship in Complementary Health care, Mitchell A & Cormack M, Churchill Livingstone, 1998

Vital Practice – Stories from the healing arts: the homeopathic and supervisory way, Ryan S. Sea Change, 2004

Websites

Liz Koch: www.coreawareness.com

Emilie Conrad's continuum work: www.continuummovement.com

The Egoscue method: www.egoscue.com

The Pilates Foundation: www.pilatesfoundation.com

Body Control Pilates: www.bodycontrol.co.uk

British Wheel of Yoga: www.bwy.org.uk

Stuart Hameroff: www.quantumconsciousness.org

The Acupuncture System and The Liquid Crystalline Collagen Fibres of the Connective Tissues

Liquid Crystalline Meridians

Mae-Wan Ho (Ph.D.) and David P. Knight (Ph.D.)

Reprint permission arranged with The Acupuncture System and the Liquid Crystalline Collagen Fibers of the Connective Tissues/, The American Journal of Chinese Medicine/, Vol. 26, Nos. 3-4 (1998). @ World Scientific Publishing, Singapore. For further details visit www.i-sis.org.uk

Abstract

We propose that the acupuncture system and the DC body field detected by Western scientists both inhere in the continuum of liquid crystalline collagen fibres that make up the bulk of the connective tissues. Bound water layers on the collagen fibres provide proton conduction pathways for rapid intercommunication throughout the body, enabling the organism to function as a coherent whole. This liquid crystalline continuum mediates hyperreactivity to allergens and the body's responsiveness to different forms of subtle energy medicine. It constitutes a "body consciousness" working in tandem with the "brain consciousness" of the nervous system. We review supporting evidence from biochemistry, cell biology, biophysics and neurophysiology, and suggest experiments to test our hypothesis.

Meridians and fields

The meridian theory is a prominent component of traditional Chinese medicine. It was formulated in ancient China with the practice of acupuncture, moxibustion, massage and qigong - an integrated mind-body exercise for controlling and mobilizaing qi (energy) for physical fitness and well-being. The meridians are a complicated system of pathways in which "qi and blood" are said to circulate in the body, thus interconnecting the viscera and limbs, the deeper and superficial layers of the body in a fine meshwork (Yin, 1992). The meridians have effectively guided diagnosis and treatment of diseases by drugs, acupuncture, moxibustion, and massage for thousands of years. Acupuncture is also widely used for pain relief, anaesthesia, and in some cases, for treating psychiatric disturbances (Esser et al, 1976).

Yet, the meridians and their acupuncture points have no known, straightforward anatomical correlates recognized in western medicine, such as the circulatory system or the nervous system. Attempts continue to be made to establish anatomical and functional connections between acupuncture points and a variety of structures. These include receptors supplied by sensory nerves (Wang and Liu, 1989), tendon organs, encapsulated nerve-endings, extensive neural terminals, vascular network or superficial blood vessels (Gunn, 1976; Pan et al, 1988), veins perforating fascia (Plummer, 1980), and mast cells (Zhai, 1988).

Since the 1970s, there has been growing interest in the electrical characteristics of acupuncture points and in developing instruments for diagnostic and therapeutic purposes, as reviewed by Tiller (1982). Such instruments all measure skin conductances and how they change on being stimulated by direct current (DC) or alternating current (AC). Measurements of DC skin conductances have provided evidence that acupuncture points and meridians have distinctive electrical properties compared with the surrounding skin. Acupuncture points typically represent local maxima in conductance, elevated by a factor of 10 to 100, compared with the surrounding skin, while acupuncture meridians have the chracteristics of electrical transmission lines (Tiller, 1973; Reichmannis et al, 1976; Becker, 1990). Tiller (1982, 1987) has presented several models to account for the electrical properties of acupuncture points based on charge movements and selective permeability of ions through different layers of the skin.

In the kind of measurement offered by Motoyama (1980), multiple fixed electrodes are positioned over 28 acupuncture points on the hands and feet, while the large reference electrode is attached to the wrist. A direct current is passed through the circuit by a 3V battery. The conductance typically shows a fast decay in microseconds, overlying a slow baseline conductance with a relaxation time of some tens of seconds. Motoyama attributes the fast component to semi-conduction in the dermis, while the slow component is attributed to ion movements and storage across the basal membrane separating the dermis from the epidermis. Tiller (1987) represents the epidermal and dermal layers as two domains in series, each with its capacitance and resistance with very different response (relaxation) times. The fast component is associated with the dermis, the low frequency component, the epidermis. Tiller has further suggested that the fast conductance might be due to H+, as the DC voltage supplied (3V) was sufficient to ionize water. This model identifies the differing electrical properties of the dermis and epidermis, which could account for some, though not all, of the responses of the acupuncture system to electrical stimulation. These responses are often found to correlate with states of disease and health (Becker et al, 1976; Kobayashi, 1985).

According to traditional theory, the acupuncture system is an active circulatory system for mobilizing energy and for intercommunication throughout the body. So, it is unlikely to be completely understood in terms of the passive responses of skin conductances to electrodermal stimulation. The most promising functional correlate of the acupuncture system, as Becker (1990) suggests, is the direct current (DC) electrodynamical field that he and others have detected in the body of all organisms. This DC body field is involved in morphogenesis during development, in wound-healing and regeneration subsequent to injury. The direct currents making up the body field are not due to charged ions but instead depend on a mode of semi-conduction characteristic of solid state systems (Becker, 1961). The acupuncture points, moreover, may act as "booster amplifiers" of the very weak currents that typically flow along the meridians.

According to Becker (1990), the DC body field is not located in the nervous sytem itself, but in "perineural" tissues such as the glial cells in the brain and spinal cord, and the schwann cells encasing the peripheral nerves. This hypothesis would seem to conflict with the suggestion that the DC body field is correlated with the acupuncture system. The acupuncture system is clearly not directly associated with the perineural tissues, although it may have functional interconnections with the central and peripheral nervous system (Gunn, 1976; Wang and Liu, 1989; Pan et al, 1988). Also, an electrodynamical field can be detected in all early embryos and in plants and animals which do not have neural or perineural tissues (Burr and Northrup, 1935). It is likely that the DC field is functionally interconnected with the nervous system, and yet exists, to a large degree, outside the nervous system. In fact, it is widely recognized that under a variety of conditions, the speed of communication in our body is much faster than can be accounted for by the known speed of nerve conduction (see Ho, 1997a), and nerves simply do not reach all parts of our body.

We propose that both the DC electrodynamical field and the acupuncture system have a common anatomical basis. It is the aligned, collagen liquid crystalline continuum in the connective tissues of the body with its layers of structured water molecules supporting rapid semi-conduction of protons. This enables all parts of the body to intercommunicate readily, so the organism can function as a coherent whole. This liquid crystalline continuum may mediate hyperreactivity to allergens and the body's responsiveness to different forms of subtle energy medicine. Furthermore, it constitutes a "body consciousness" that is functionally interconnected with the "brain consciousness" of the nervous system (Ho, 1997a). We review supporting evidence from biochemistry, cell biology, biophysics and neurophysiology, and suggest experiments to test our hypothesis.

The organism is a liquid crystalline continuum

One requirement for an intercommunication system is a continuum which can carry the signals for intercommunication.

For example, a continuum of air, liquid or solid, can all serve as medium for sound and mechanical waves. If the medium is electrically polarizable, it will also transmit polarization waves. Electromagnetic waves are thought to be an exception, as they can travel through empty space. But to this day, physicists are still debating the nature of the vacuum, which carries not only electromagnetic waves but also gravity waves (see Laszlo, 1995). The living organism is a continuum. Not only is the entire cell now known to be mechanically and electrically interconnected in a "solid state" (Clegg and Drost-Hansen, 1991) or "tensegrity system" (Ingber, 1993, 1998); all the cells in the body are in turn interconnected to one another via the connective tissues (Oschman, 1984, 1996). More accurately, perhaps, we recently discovered that the living continuum is liquid crystalline, with all the properties that make liquid crystals ideal for intercommunication (Ho et al, 1996; Ho, 1997a).

Liquid crystals are states or phases of matter in between solid crystals and liquids, hence the term, mesophases. Unlike liquids which have little or no molecular order, liquid crystals have orientational order, and varying degrees of translational order. But unlike solid crystals, liquid crystals are flexible, malleable, and responsive (De Gennes, 1974; Collings, 1990). There are many kinds of liquid crystals, from those which are most like liquids, to ones that most resemble solid crystals. Those that are like liquids can flow in the way water does, and even though all molecules tend to be aligned in one direction, individual molecules can move quite freely and change places with one another while maintaining their common orientation. The ones that resemble solid crystals will have order in all three dimensions, and molecules may even be extensively covalently cross-linked together, but they will remain flexible and responsive.

Liquid crystals typically undergo rapid changes in orientation or phase transitions when exposed to electric (and magnetic) fields - which is why they are widely used in display screens. They also respond to changes in temperature, hydration, shear forces and pressure. Biological liquid crystals carry static electric charges and are therefore also influenced by pH, salt concentration and dielectric constant of the solvent (Collings, 1990; Knight and Feng, 1993). George Gray (1993), who has studied liquid crystals for many years, refers to liquid crystals as "tunable responsive systems", and as such, ideal for making organisms.

It is already widely recognized that all the major constituents of living organisms may be liquid crystalline (Collings, 1990) - lipids of cellular membranes, DNA, possibly all proteins, especially cytoskeletal proteins, muscle proteins, and proteins in the connective tissues such as collagens and proteoglycans (Bouligand, 1972; Giraud-Guille, 1992; Knight and Feng, 1993). Recent nuclear magnetic resonance (nmr) studies of muscles in living human subjects provide evidence of their "liquid-crystalline-like" structure (Kreis and Boesch, 1994). However, very few workers have yet come to grips with the idea that organisms may be essentially liquid crystalline.

The importance of liquid crystals for living organization was actually recognized a long time ago, as pointed out by Joseph Needham (1935). Hardy suggested in 1927 that molecular orientation may be important for living protoplasm, and Peters, two years later, made the explicit link between molecular orientation and liquid crystals. Needham, indeed, proposed that organisms actually are liquid crystalline. But direct evidence for that has only recently been provided by Ho and coworkers (Ho and Lawrence, 1993; Ho and Saunders, 1994; Ho et al, 1996), who successfully imaged live organisms using an interference colour technique that amplifies weak birefringences typical of biological liquid crystals. They further discover that all organisms so far examined are polarized along the anterior-posterior or oral-adoral axis, so that when that axis is properly aligned, all the tissues in the body are maximally coloured; the colours changing in concert as the organism is rotated from that position. Not only live organisms, but also fresh-frozen or well-fixed sections of the skin, cartilage and tendons, all exhibit the same brilliant interference colours typical of living organisms.

The connective tissues are still regarded by most workers in purely mechanical terms - their functions are to keep the body in shape, to act as packing between the major organs and tissues, to strengthen the wall of arteries, veins, intestines and air passages, and to provide the rigid elements (bony skeleton) for the attachment of muscles. A more enlightened view is that of a global tensegrity system, in which compression elements (bones) are interconnected with tension elements (muscles, tendons and ligaments), and local stimuli invariably lead to global reorganization of the whole (Ingber, 1998).

Actually, connective tissues may also be largely responsible for the rapid intercommunication that enables our body to function effectively as a coherent whole, and are therefore central to our health and well-being.

Collagens and Intercommunication

The clue to the intercommunication function of connective tissues lies in the properties of collagen, which makes up 70% or more of all the protein of the connective tissues. Connective tissues, in turn form the bulk of the body of most multicellular animals. Collagen is therefore the most abundant protein in the animal kingdom (Knight and Feng, 1993).

There are many kinds of collagens, all sharing a general repeating sequence of the tripeptide, (gly-X-Y) - where X and Y are usually proline or hydroxyproline. They also share a molecular structure in which three polypeptide chains are wound around one another in a triple-helix, with the compact amino acid glycine in the central axis of the helix, while the bulky amino-acids proline and hydroxyproline are near the surface (Van der Rest and Garrone, 1991). In the fibrous forms, the triple-helical molecules aggregate head to tail and side-by side into long fibrils, and bundles of fibrils in turn assemble into thicker fibres, and other more complex three-dimensional liquid crystalline structures. Some collagens assemble into sheets constructed from an open, liquid crystalline meshwork of molecules. All these structures are formed by self-assembly, in the sense that they need no specific "instructions" other than certain conditions of pH, ionic strength, temperature and hydration. The process seems to be predominantly driven by hydrophilic interactions due to hydrogen-bonding between water molecules and charged amino-acid side-chains (Leikin et al, 1995). However, the precise mesophase structures resulting from different conditions of self-assembly show endless variations (Zhou et al, 1996; Haffegee et al, 1998). The different kinds of collagen assemblies in different connective tissues are generally well-suited to the mechanical tasks performed by the connective tissue concerned, because they were shaped by the prevailing conditions and the relevant mechanical forces.

Recent studies reveal that collagens are not just materials with mechanical properties. Instead, they have dielectric and electrical conductive properties that make them very sensitive to mechanical pressures, pH, and ionic composition (Leikin et al, 1993, 1995), and to electromagnetic fields. The electrical properties depend, to a large extent, on the bound water molecules in and around the collagen triple-helix. X-ray diffraction studies reveal a cylinder of water surrounding the triple-helix which is hydrogen-bonded to the hydroxyproline side-chains (Bella et al, 1994). Nuclear magnetic resonance studies have provided evidence of three populations of water molecules associated with collagen. These are interstitial water, very tightly bound within the triple helix of the collagen molecule, and strongly interacting with the peptide bonds of the polypeptide chains; bound water, corresponding to the more loosely structured water-cylinder on the surface of the triple helix; and free water filling the spaces between the fibrils and between fibres (Peto and Gillis, 1990).Evidence for bound water in collagen also comes from studies using another popular physical measurement technique, Fourier Transform Infra Red (FTIR) spectroscopy (Renugopalakrishnan et al, 1989).

Bound water, or vicinal water is a very general phenomenon involving the structuring of water on solid surfaces. It is already known that up to 50 or 60% of the cell water is structured in the enormous "microtrabecular lattice" that fills the entire cell (Clegg and Drost-Hansen, 1991), which gives the cell its "solid-state" like characteristic (see above).

The existence of the ordered network of water molecules, connected by hydrogen bonds, and interspersed within the protein fibrillar matrix of the collagens is especially signicant, as it is expected to support rapid jump conduction of protons - positive electric charges - and this has been confirmed by dielectric measurements (Sasaki, 1984). The conductivity of collagen increases strongly with the amount of water absorbed (from 0.1 to 0.3g/g of dry collagen), in accordance with the power-law relation, $\sigma(\emptyset) = X\emptyset Y$ where $\emptyset$ is the water content, and X and Y are constants. The value of Y is found to be 5.1 to 5.4, and is a function of the collagen fibrillar structure. These results suggest that continuous chains of ordered water molecules join neighbouring ion-generating sites enabling proton jumps to occur. The high value of the exponential suggests that up to 5 or 6 neighbours may be involved in the jump conduction. Based on these findings, it is estimated that conductivity along the collagen fibres is at least one-hundred times that across the fibre (Pethig, 1996). Measurements have yet to be made to reveal the true extent of anisotropy in conductivity. The increase in conductivity is most marked around 310 K (Jaroszyk and Marzec, 1993), which interestingly, is close to the normal temperature of our body. It is to be noted that the triple-helix of collagens in dilute solutions "melt" at around the same temperature - 40°C (Leikin et al, 1995). Melting may enable the collagen fibres to better realign, and hence increase conductivity. Collagen melting and realignment may be one of contributing factors to the now well-documented health-promoting effects of physical exercise (see Bortz, 1996).

The collagenous liquid crystalline mesophases in the connective tissues, with their associated structured water, therefore, constitutes a semi-conducting, highly responsive network that extends throughout the organism. This network is directly linked to the intracellular matrices of individual cells via proteins that go through the cell membrane. The connective tissues and intracellular matrices, together, form a global tensegrity system (Oschman, 1984; Ingber, 1998), as well as an excitable electrical continuum for rapid intercommunication throughout the body (Ho, 1997a).

Collagen fibre orientation and the acupuncture system

A major factor contributing to the efficiency of intercommunication is the structured, oriented nature of collagen liquid crystalline mesophases in all connective tissues. Each connective tissue has its characteristic orientation of fibrous structures which are clearly related to the mechanical stresses and strains to which the tissue is subject. This same orientation may also be crucial for intercommunication. Collagen alignment has long been recognized to be important in the structure of bone and cartilage. Less well known are the "Langer lines" (Langer, 1978) in the skin, corresponding to predominant orientations of collagen fibres, which are determined, at least in part, by stresses during development and growth (Reihsner et al, 1995).

Collagen fibre alignments in connective tissues providing channels for electrical intercommunication may thus be correlated with the acupuncture system of meridians and points in traditional Chinese medicine, which, as mentioned above, is also related to the DC body field identified by scientists in the West.

As collagen fibres are expected to conduct (positive) electricity preferentially along the fibres due to the bound water, which are predominantly oriented along the fibre axis; it follows that these conduction paths may correspond to acupuncture meridians. By contrast, acupuncture points typically exibit low electrical resistances compared with the surrounding skin, and may therefore correspond to singularities or gaps between collagen fibres, or, where collagen fibres are oriented at right angles to the dermal layer. A number of structures mentioned earlier, which are at or near acupuncture points, have a common feature in that they are located in local gaps in the fascia or collagen fibres (see Meridians and Fields). Actual conducting channels may bear a more subtle relationship to the orientation of the collagen fibres, as conductivity depends predominantly on the layer(s) of bound water on the surface of the collagen molecules rather than the collagens themselves. So-called free water may also take part in proton conduction as the result of induced polarization, particularly as water molecules naturally form hydrogen-bonded networks (Luzar and Chandler, 1996). This would be consistent with the observed increase in conductivity of collagen as hydration increases to a level well beyond the bound water fraction, around 0.15g/g dry weight; and also with the fact that the normal hydration level of tendon is about 65%.

That conductive pathways actually link the entire body is demonstrated by Han Wan and Robert Balaban of the Canadian National Heart, Lung and Blood Institute (see Ehrenstein, 1997), who are taking advantage of the variation in conductivity of different layers of tissues in the body to develop a new, non-destructive imaging technique to aid clinical diagnosis.

The correlation between collagen alignment and the acupuncture system could be tested by examining the alignment in skin biopsies at acupuncture points and meridians - with corroborative skin conductance measurements - compared with non-acupuncture, non-merdian areas. In this connection, we have developed a quantitative imaging package based on our interference colour polarizing microscopy that readily plots molecular alignment in sections of the skin and other connective tissues (Knight et al, 1996; Ross et al, 1997).

Collagen alignment in health and injury

If our hypothesis is correct, and patterns of collagen fibre alignment are indeed important for intercommunication, then they would be expected to affect the health of the individuals concerned, and also to be involved in the processes of healing and regeneration.

Electrical injury currents typically flow from skin wounds and sites of amputation, which are found to be involved in healing and regeneration (Becker, 1990). Injury currents themselves constitute evidence that conductive circuits link the entire body, so that cuts result in leakage currents. The leakage currents mobilize cells to migrate to the site of injury to initiate the healing and regenerative processes. It is significant that the immediate injury currents are all positive, as suggestive of proton currents. Only later on, after the regenerating blastema is formed, do the currents reverse to negative (see Becker, 1990).

Since these observations were made, electromagnetic interventions have been widely used for stimulating regeneration or healing, with conflicting results. Part of the problem may have been that the strengths of electromagnetic fields used were far stronger than the endogenous fields. Another important factor which has received little attention may be the orientation of the applied electromagnetic field with respect to the alignment of collagen fibres at the site of injury. If the field orientation is inappropriate, then application of the external field is likely to be ineffective, and may even delay recovery (Watkins et al, 1985).On the basis of the estimated 100-fold difference in electrical conductivity along the fibre compared to that across the fibre, it would be expected that collagens fibres will align in the direction of the applied electric field. Again these experiments should be done to ascertain the optimum conditions for collagen alignments, which may have important implications for healing and regeneration.

Oriented Collagens and Body consciousness

Proteins in liquid crystals have coherent motions, in the first place, because the molecules are aligned, so that not all the degrees of freedom of movement that individual molecules have will be available in the liquid crystal mesophase (Searle and Williams, 1992). Protein motions involve vibrational deformations of peptide bonds, which will generate polarization waves along the proteins, accompanied by proton conduction in the structured water shell. Fröhlich (1980) has predicted that coherent vibrations (or excitations) will result from metabolic pumping in dielectric systems such as organisms, where electromagnetic and electromechanical forces are expected to interact. Liquid crystallinity will make coherent excitations even more likely to happen. Weak signals of mechanical pressure, heat or electricity, may therefore be readily amplified and propagated by a modulation of the proton currents or coherent polarization waves (Mikhailov and Ert, 1996)

The hydrogen-bonded water network of the connective tissues is actually linked to ordered water dipoles in the ion-channels of the cell membrane that allow inorganic ions to pass in and out of the cell (Williams, 1993). There is thus a direct electrical link between distant signals and the intracellular matrix, leading to physiological changes inside the cells, including neurons and glial cells. This electrical channel of intercommunication is in addition to, and coupled with, the mechanical tensegrity interactions of the connective tissue-intracellular matrix continuum mentioned above. Any mechanical deformations of the protein-bound water network will automatically result in electrical disturbances and conversely, electrical disturbances will result in mechanical effects. The new imaging technique that Han and Balaban are developing (see above) depends specifically on detecting ultrasound emissions from mechanoelastic vibrations caused by electrical pulses applied to the tissues.

Proton jump-conduction is a form of semi-conduction in condensed matter, and is much faster than conduction of electrical signals by the nerves. Thus the 'ground substance' of the entire body may provide a much better intercom munication system than the nervous system. Indeed, it is possible that one of the functions of the nervous system is to slow down intercommunication through the ground substance. Lower animals which do not have a nervous system are nonetheless sensitive. At the other end of the evolutionary scale, note the alarming speed with which a hypersensitive response occurs in human beings. There is no doubt that a body consciousness exists prior to the "brain" consciousness associated with the nervous system. This body consciousness also has a memory, as argued in the section following.

Crystal Memory

Many studies on the conformation (three-dimensional shape) of the collagen triple-helix have shown that subtle changes are correlated with specific biological activities (Fields, 1995). Cells are guided in their growth and movement by contact with collagens, and specific sites are recognized by a host of cell membrane proteins. Mutations altering collagen amino-acid sequences give subtle changes in the conformation (Bella et al, 1994) which are associated with hereditary diseases, such as osteogenesis imperfecta, chondrodysplasias and Ehler-Danlos syndrome. Changes in collagen conformation should alter the bound water. Conformations of proteins are by no means static. All proteins undergo a hierarchy of conformational changes on a range of timescales, and collagens are unlikely to be exceptions. The conformations are clustered in groups of nearly identical energy content, with very low energy barriers between individual members of the group, but separated from other groups by higher energy barriers (see Welch, 1985). Collective changes in conformation (or phase transitions) can readily be triggered, in turn altering the liquid crystalline structure and the bound water network, as dielectric studies on synthetic liquid crystals have documented (Leikin et al, 1993; Wrobel et al, 1988).

As the collagens and bound water form a global network, there will be a certain degree of stability, or resistance to change. This constitutes a memory, which may be further stabilized by cross-linking and other chemical modifications of the collagens. The network will retain tissue memory of previous experiences, but it will also have the capacity to register new experiences, as all connective tissues, including bones, are not only constantly intercommunicating and responsive, but also undergo metabolic turnover like the rest of our body. Memory is thus dynamically distributed in the structured network and the associated, self-reinforcing circuits of proton currents, the sum total of which will be expected to make up the DC body field itself.

Coupled Body and Brain Consciousness

We have argued that a body consciousness possessing all the hallmarks of consciousness - sentience, intercommunication and memory - is distributed throughout the entire body. Brain consciousness associated with the nervous system is embedded in body consciousness and is coupled to it (see also Ho, 1997a,b; 1998). That bound water plays a crucial role in conscious experience is supported by recent evidence that anaesthetics act by replacing and releasing bound water from proteins and membrane interfaces, thus destroying the hydrogen-bonded network that can support proton jump-conduction (Tsukamoto and Oglie, 1995).Significantly, Becker (1990) found that general anaesthesia also leads to the complete attenuation of the DC body field. It would be of interest to study the conductivities of collagen equilibrated with different solvents and anaesthetics. We would predict that collagens equilibrated with anaethetics will show a decrease in conductivity compared to an equivalently hydrated sample.

Although brain and body consciousness are normally coupled to each other, they may decouple under certain circumstances. Surgical patients under general anaesthesia have been known to regain (brain) consciousness of pain, but not the ability to move or to express their distress. In contrast, acupuncture has been successfully used to anaesthesize patients who are fully awake. Further evidence that brain and body consciousness are to some extent independent is Becker's (1990) observation that during a perceptive event, local changes in the DC field can be measured half a second before sensory signals arrive in the brain. Similarly, Libet et al (1979) produced evidence suggesting that a "readiness potential" precedes the decision of a subject to move an arm or a leg. It appears that the activities in the brain may be preconditioned by the local DC field.

If it is true that brain and body consciousness can decouple from one another, it would be important to develop monitoring systems specific to either of them. For example, acupuncture points may show changes independently of the EEG, and hence, surgical patients whose EEG, or better yet, whose magnetoencephalogram (MEG) measured with the ultrasensitive SQUID magnetometer show wakefulness may yet have acupuncture point(s) electrodermal readings typical of the anaesthetized state. Similarly, patients anaethetized by acupuncture should have the appropriate "anaethetized" electrodermal readings even though their EEG or MEG is fully "awake".

Conclusion

We have proposed that the acupuncture (meridian) system and the DC body field detected by Western scientists both inhere in the continuum of liquid crystalline collagen fibres and the associated layers of bound water that make up the bulk of the connective tissues of the body. Acupuncture merdians may be associated with the bound water layers along oriented collagen fibres, which provide proton conduction pathways for rapid intercommunication throughout the body; while acupuncture points may correspond to gaps in the fibres or fibres oriented at right angles to the surface of the skin. The sum total of the electrical and electromechanical activities of the liquid crystalline continuum constitutes a "body consciousness" that works in tandem with the "brain consciousness" of the nervous system. We have reviewed supporting evidence from biochemistry, cell biology, biophysics and neurophysiology, and have suggested the following experiments to test our hypothesis.

1.   Dielectric measurements on oriented samples of collagen fibres, to ascertain the anisotropy of conductivity along and across the fibres.
2.   Dielectric measurements on the conductivities of oriented samples of collagen fibres equilibrated with different anaesthetics, to ascertain the decrease in conductivity compared with samples equilibrated with water (see p. 13).
3.   Examination of collagen fibre alignments in skin biopsies at acupuncture points and meridians - with corroborative skin conductance measurements - compared with non-acupuncture, non-meridian areas. This is to ascertain the association of meridians with oriented fibres and acupoints with gaps or with fibres oriented at right angles to the surface of the skin.
4.   Alignment of collagen fibres in the direction of an applied electric field, predicted from the anisotropy in electrical conductivity along and across the fibre.
5.   Simultaneous measurements of EEG/MEG and skin conductances of acupuncture points of patients under chemical anaesthesia to detect correlated and uncorrelated activities between brain and body consciousness.
6.   Simultaneous measurements of EEG/MEG and skin conductances of acupuncture points of patients under acupuncture anaesthesia to detect possible uncorrelated activities between brain and body consciousness.

It is reasonable to conclude that under normal, healthy conditions, body and brain consciousness mutually inform and condition each other, and that the unity of our conscious experience and our state of health depends on the complete coherence of brain and body. Traditional Chinese medicine based on the acupuncture meridian system places the emphasis of health on the coherence of body functions which harmonizes brain to body, which makes perfect sense if one recognizes the brain as part of the body. Western medicine, by contrast, has yet no concept of the whole, and is based, at the very outset, on a Cartesian divide between mind and brain, and brain and body.

References

1. Becker, R.O. Proof that the direct electrical currents in the salamander are semiconducting innature. Science 134, 101-102, 1961.

2. Becker, R.O. Cross Currents. The Promise of Electromedicine, the Perils of Electropollution. Jeremy P. Tarcher, Inc., Los Angeles, 1990.

3. Becker, R., M. Reichmanis and A. Marino. Electrophysiological correlates of acupuncture points and meridians. Psychoenergetic Systems 1: 105, 1976.

4. Bella, J., M. Eaton, B.Brodsky and H.M. Berman. Crystal and molecular structure of a collagen-like peptide at 1.9Å resolution. Science 266, 75-81, 1994.

5. Bouligand, Y. Twisted Fibrous Arrangement in Biological Materials and Cholesteric Mesophases. Tissue and Cell 4, 189-217, 1972.

6. Bortz, W. Dare to be 100, Simon and Schuster, New York, 1996.

7. Burr, H.S. and F.S.C. Northrup. The electro-dynamic theory of life. Quart. Rev. Biol. 10: 322-333, 1935.

8. Clegg, J.S. and W. Drost-Hansen. On the biochemistry and cell physiology of water. In Biochemistry and Molecular Biology of Fishes, Vol 1, pp. 1-23, Elsevier Science Publisher, Amsterdam, 1991.

9. Collings, P.J. Liquid Crystals, Nature's Delicate Phase of Matter, Princeton University Press, Princeton, 1990.

10. De Gennes, P.G. The Physics of Liquid Crystals, Clarendon Press, Oxford, 1974.

11. Ehrenstein, D. New technique maps the body electric. Science 176: 681, 1997.

12. Esser, A.H., S.T. Botek and C.G. Gilbert. Acupuncture tonification: adjunct in psychia tricrehabilitation. American Journal of Chinese Medicine 4: 73-79, 1976.

13. Fields, G.B. The collagen triple-helix: correlation of conformation with biological activities. Connective Tissue Research 31: 235-243, 1995.

14. Fröhlich, H. The biological effects of microwaves and related questions. Adv. Electronics and Electron. Phys. 53: 85-152, 1980.

15. Giraud-Guille, M.M. Liquid crystallinity in condensed type I collagen solutions. A clue to the packing of collagen in extracellular matrices. Journal of Molecular Biology 224: 861-873, 1992.

16. Gray, G. Liquid crystals - molecular self-assembly. British Association for the Advancement of Science, chemistry Session: Molecular Self-assembly in Science and Life, Presidential Address, Keele, U.K., 1993.

17. Gunn, C.C. Acupncture loci, a proposal for their classification according to their Relationship to known neural structures. Am. J. Clin. Med. 4: 183-195, 1976.

18. Haffegee, J., M.W. Ho and Y.M. Zhou, unpublished results, 1998.

19. Ho, M.W. Quantum Coherence and Conscious Experience. Kybernetes, 26: 265-276, 1997a.

20. Ho, M.W. Towards a theory of the organism. Integrative Physiological and Behavioral Science 32: 1997b.

21. Ho, M.W. The Rainbow and the Worm, The Physics of Organisms, 2nd ed., World Scientific, Singapore, 1998.

22. Ho, M.W., Haffegee J., Newton, R., Zhou, Y.M., Bolton, J.S., Ross, S.: Organisms as polyphasic liquid crystals. Bioelectrochemistry and Bioenergetics 41, 81-91, 1996.

23. Ho, M.W., Lawrence, M. Interference Colour Vital Imaging: A Novel Noninvasive Microsopic Technique. Microscopy and Analysis September, 26.

24. Ho, M.W. and P.T. Saunders. Liquid crystalline mesophases in living organisms. in Bioelectrodynamics and Biocommunication, Ho, M.W., F.A. Popp and U. Warnke (Eds.), World Scientific, Singapore, 1994.

25. Ingber, D.E. The riddle of morphogenesis: a question of solution chemistry or molecular cell engineering? Cell 75: 1249-1252, 1993.

26. Ingber, D.E. The architecture of life. Scientific American January: 48-57, 1998.

27. Jaroszyk, F. and E. Marze. Dielectric properties of BAT collagen in the temperature range of thermalcenaturation. Ber. Bunsenges. Phys. Chem. 97: 868-872, 1993.

28. Knight, D. and D. Feng. Collagens as liquid crystals. Paper presented in British Association for the Advancement of Science, Chemistry Session, Molecular Self-Assembly in Science and Life, Keele, 1993.

29. Knight, D.P., S.W. Hu, L.J. Gathercole, M. Rusaöuen-Innocent, M.W. Ho and R. Newton, Molecular orientation in an extruded collagenous composite, the marginal rib of the egg capsule of the dogfish Cyliorhinus canicula: a novel lyotropic liquid crystalline arrangement and how it is defined in the spinneret. Philos. Trans. R. Soc. London 351: 1205-1232, 1996.

30. Kobayashi, T. Early diagnosis of microcancer by cancer check of related acupuncture meridian. American Journal of Acupuncture 13: 63-68, 1985.

31. Kreis, R., Boesch, C. Liquid-crystal-like structure of human muscle demonstrated by in vivo observation of direct dipolar coupling in localized proton magnetic resonance spectroscopy. Journal of Magnetic Resonance B 104: 189-192, 1994.

32. Langer, K. On the anatomy and physiology of the skin. British Journal of Plastic Surgery 31: 3-8, 1978.

33. Laszlo, E. The Interconnected Universe, World Scientific, Singapore, 1995.

34. Leikin, S., V.A. Parsegian, D.C. Rau and R.P. Rand. Hydration forces. Ann. Rev. Phys. Chem. 44: 369-395, 1993.

35. Leikin, S., D.C. Rau and V.A. Parsegian. Temperature-favoured assembly of collagen is driven by hydrophilic not hydrophobic interactions. Structural Biology 2: 205-210, 1995.

36. Libet, B., E.W. Wright, Jr., B. Feinstein and D.K. Pearl. Subjective referral of the timing for a conscious sensory experience. Brain 102: 193-224, 1979.

37. Luzar, A. and D. Chandler. Hydrogen-bond kinetics in liquid water. Nature 379: 55-57, 1996.

38. Mikhailov, A.S., Ertl, G.: Nonequilibrium Structures in Condensed Systems. Science 272: 1596-1597, 1996.

39. Motoyama, H. Electrophysiological and preliminary biochemical studies of skin properties in relation to the acupuncture meridian. International Association for Religion and Parapsychology 6: 1-36, 1980.

40. Needham, J. Order and Life, Yale University Press, New Haven, 1935.

41. Oschman, J.L. Structure and properties of ground substances. American Zoologist 24: 199 215, 1984.

42. Oschman, J.L. A Biophysical Basis of Acupuncture, Private manuscript, 1993.

43. Pan, C. and A. Zhao. in Research on Acupuncture, Moxibustion and Acupuncture Anesthesia, Shang, X. (Ed.) Springer-Verlag, New York, 1988.

44. Peto, S. and P. Gillis. Fiber-to-field angle dependence of proton nuclear magnetic relaxation in collagen. Magnetic Resonance Imaging 8: 703-712, 1990.

45. Plummer, J.P. Anatomical finding at acupuncture loci. Am. J. Clin. Med. 8: 170-180, 1980.

46. Reichmannis, M., A.A. Marion and R.O. Becker. D.C. skin conductance variation at acupuncture loci. American Journal of Chinese Medicine 4: 69-72, 1976.

47. Reihsner, R., B. Balogh and E.J. Menzel. Two-dimensional elastic properties of human skin in terms of an incremental model at the in vivo configuration. Med. Eng. Phy. 17: 304-313, 1995.

48. Renugopalakrishnan, V., G. Chandrakasan, S. Moore, T.B. Hutson, C.V. Berney and R.S. Bhatnagar. Bound water in collagen. Evidence from Fourier Transform Infrared and Fourier Transform Infrared Photoacoustic Spectroscopic study. Macromolecules 22: 4121-4124, 1989.

49. Ross, S., R. Newton, Y.M. Zhou, H. Jaffegee, M.W. Ho, J.P. Bolton and D. Knight. Quantitative image analysis of birefringent biological material. Journal of Microscopy 187: 62-67, 1997.

50. Sasaki, N. Dielectric properties of slightly hydrated collagen. time-water content superposition analysis. Biopolymers 23: 1725-1734, 1984.

51. Searle, M.S. and D.H. Williams. The cost of conformation order: entropy changes in molecular associations. Journal of American Chemical Society 114: 10690-10697, 1992.

52. Tiller, W.A. Explanation of electrodermal diagnostic and treatment instruments: Part I. Electrical behavior of human skin. Journal of Holistic Medicine 4: 105-127, 1982.

53. Tiller, W.A. Some energy field observations of man and nature, in Galaxies of Life, Krippner, S. and D. Rubin (Ed.), New York, Interface, 1973.

54. Tiller, W.A. What do electrodermal diagnostic acupuncture instruments really measure. American Journal of Acupuncture 15(1), 18-23, 1987.

55. Tsukamoto, I. and K. Ogli. Effects of anesthetics on the interfacial polarity of membranes - evaluated by Taft's polarity parameters. Prog. Anesth. Mech. 3: 368-373, 1995.

56. Van der Rest, M. and R. Garrone. Collagen family of proteins. FASEB 5: 2814-2823, 1991.

57. Wang, K. and J. Liu. Needling sensation receptor of an acupoint supplied by the median nerve - studies of their electro-physiological characteristics. American Journal of Chinese Medicine 17: 145-155, 1989.

58. Watkins, J.P., J.A. Auer, S.J. Morgans and S. Gay. Healing of surgically created defects in the equine superficial digitalflexor tendon: effect of pulsing electromagnetic field therapy on collagen-type transformation and tissue morphologic reorganization. American Journal of Veterinary Research 46: 2097-2103, 1985.

59. Welch, G.R. Organized Multienzyme Systems, Academic Press, Orlando, 1985.

60. Williams, R.J.P. The history of the proton-driven ATP formation. Bioscience Reports 13: 191-212, 1993.

61. Wrobel, S., B. Gestblom, E. Noreland and J.S. Doane. Dielectric relaxation of water molecules in different lyotropic structures of nonylphenoxypoly (ethylenoxy) ethanol. Liquid Crystals 3: 825-832, 1988.

62. Yin, H. Fundamentals of Traditional Chinese Medicine. Beijing: Foreign Language Press, 1992.

63. Zhai, N. Research on the histophysiological relation of mastocytes and meridians (Chinese). Clin. Acupunt. Moxibust. 8: 50-53, 1988.

64. Zhou, Y.M., R.H. Newton, J. Haffegee, J.Y. Brown, S. Ross, J.P. Bolton and M.W. Ho. Imaging liquid crystalline mesophases in vivo and in vitro: measuring molecular birefringence and order parameter of liquid crystals. Bios Journal, 1996.

Biography

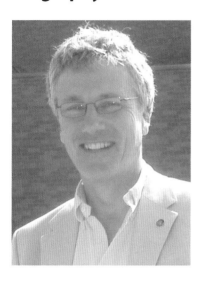

John Wilks MA FRSA RCST BTAA

After studying music at Oxford University, John developed a strong interest in body-orientated psychotherapy and meditation. He has been practising the Bowen Technique and Craniosacral Therapy full time since 1995, and works at a physiotherapy and integrated healthcare practice in the west of England.

He is a former chairman of the Bowen Association of the UK, the Craniosacral Therapy Association of the UK and the Cranial Forum, the lead body established to oversee the implementation of national standards of practice for the profession in the UK. He is a former examiner for the University of Oxford examinations board and is advisor on education and training for the Bowen Forum under the Prince of Wales' Foundation for Integrated Health.

He was accredited by the Bowen Therapy Academy of Australia to teach the Bowen Technique in 1999 and has since then taught in many countries throughout the world including Denmark, Sweden, Norway, Israel, USA, Australia, Portugal, Canada, Kuwait, El Salvador, Ireland, Austria and Germany. He was awarded a lifetime membership of the Bowen Therapy Academy of Australia in 2004.

In 2005 he set up a 2 year practitioner training for midwives in Craniosacral Therapy at Poole Hospital NHS Trust, the first of its kind to be accredited with the Royal College of Midwives.

He has been involved in a number of charitable projects organising therapeutic work overseas, including after the war in Bosnia and currently El Salvador. He is an Associate of the Royal College of Music, regularly plays in concerts in the south west of England and in 2005 was awarded a prestigious fellowship of the Royal Society of Arts.

In June 2007 he was featured in Tatler's guide to Britain's 250 best private doctors and has recently been asked to be module leader for the foundation degree course in complementary therapies at Worcester University which will feature the Bowen Technique and Craniosacral Therapy.

Quotes from people who have attended John's seminars

"I have learned more from these two days than from the six modules in terms of practical help. I know I will have many more satisfied clients now."

"Fantastic explanation how and why Bowen works and how to find the most effective procedure according to testing."

"Excellent content – a more 'scientific' approach to how Bowen works speaks to me – very well presented."

"Thank you very much for providing such a knowledgeable and wonderful teacher for the course. I have learned so much that I can apply to my practice. Bowen is the best."

Research References

Whitaker J : *The Bowen Technique: a gentle hands-on healing method that affects the autonomic nervous system as measured by heart rate variability and clinical assessment.* Paper presented at the American Academy of Environmental Medicine meeting - La Jolla, California, December 1997. The full report can be obtained from the AHEF, PO BOX 29874 , Dallas TX 75229

Dr Bernie Carter: *Evaluation of Bowen Technique in the Treatment of Frozen Shoulder.* University of Central Lancashire. Reviewed in Complementary Therapies in Medicine 01/032

Seba D : *The Bowen Technique - a potential treatment for fibromyalgia.* Paper presented as above and available from the same source.

Pritchard A : *The psychophysiological effects of the Bowen Technique.* Department of Psychphysiology, Melbourne Swinburne University, Australia 1993.

Norman A : *The Bowen Technique : a study of its prevalence and effectiveness.* University of North Carolina at Chapel Hill, Dept. of Physical Education, Exercise and Sports Science, 1998

thebowentechnique
the inside story